# ETHICS

## Contemporary challenges in health and social care

Edited by Audrey Leathard and Susan McLaren

First published in Great Britain in 2007 by

The Policy Press
University of Bristol
Fourth Floor
Beacon House
Queen's Road
Bristol BS8 1QU
UK

Tel +44 (0)117 331 4054
Fax +44 (0)117 331 4093
e-mail tpp-info@bristol.ac.uk
www.policypress.org.uk

British Library Cataloguing in Publication Data
A catalogue record for this book is available from the British Library.

Library of Congress Cataloging-in-Publication Data
A catalog record for this book has been requested.

ISBN 978 1 86134 755 8 paperback
ISBN 978 1 86134 756 5 hardcover

Cover design by Qube Design Associates, Bristol.
Printed and bound in Great Britain by MPG Books Ltd, Bodmin.

# Contents

# List of tables, figures and boxes

## Tables

## Figures

## Box

# List of contributors

**Brenda Almond**, Emeritus Professor of Moral and Social Philosophy, University of Hull, UK

Dr **Keith Andrews**, Director of the Institute of Neuropalliative Rehabilitation, Royal Hospital for Neuro-disability, London, UK

Dr **Charles Campion-Smith**, General Practitioner, Dorchester, Dorset, UK

**Mary Dombeck**, Professor, School of Nursing, University of Rochester, New York, US

**Jeff Girling**, Visiting Fellow, Manchester Business School, Manchester, UK

Dr **Jon Glasby**, Reader, and Head of Health and Social Care Partnerships at the Health Services Management Centre, University of Birmingham, UK

**David Hodgson**, Principal Lecturer in Social Work, Faculty of Health and Social Care Sciences, Kingston University, London, UK

**Robert Irvine**, Honorary Lecturer, University of Sydney, Australia

**Audrey Leathard**, Visiting Professor in Interprofessional Studies, London South Bank University, London, UK

Dr **Helen Lester**, Professor of Primary Care, University of Manchester, UK

**Emily McKie**, Associate Director for Joint Mental Health Commissioning, Lewisham, London, UK

**Susan McLaren**, Director of the Centre for Leadership and Practice Innovation and Professor of Nursing, Faculty of Health and Social Care, London South Bank University, London, UK

**John McPhee**, Associate, Legal Academic Centre, University of Sydney, Australia

**Jill Manthorpe**, Professor of Social Work, Co-Director of the Social Care Workforce Research Unit, King's College London, UK

Dr **Tobie Hittle Olsan**, Associate Professor of Clinical Nursing, Director of Education Research, School of Nursing, University of Rochester, New York, US

**Bridget Penhale**, Senior Lecturer in Gerontology, School of Nursing and Midwifery, University of Sheffield, UK

Dr **Elaine Pierce**, Head of Research and Development Support Unit, Royal Hospital for Neuro-disability, London, UK

**Clive Seale**, Professor of Sociology, Department of Human Sciences, Brunel University, UK

**Robert Stanley**, Senior Lecturer in Ethics, Healthcare Management and Research, Kingston University, London, UK

Dr **Martin Stevens**, Research Fellow, Social Care Workforce Research Unit, King's College London, UK

Dr **Louise Terry**, Senior Lecturer in Ethics and Law, London South Bank University, London, UK

**Anthea Tinker**, Professor of Social Gerontology, King's College London, UK

Dr **Colin Whittington**, Learning and Development Consultant, Bromley, London, UK

**Margaret Whittington**, Group Manager, Adult and Community Services, London Borough of Bromley, UK

# ONE

# Introduction

*Audrey Leathard and Susan McLaren*

## Summary

The aim of this publication is to show the importance of ethics in health and social care. The emphasis in both arenas of care is significant as, up to now, ethical issues have tended to focus on either health or social care separately. This chapter begins by briefly setting out definitions of ethics, followed by providing a policy overview to illustrate the increasing impact of ethics overall that has led to ever more media coverage. Summaries of the chosen topic areas are then set out where three key arenas have been assembled for discussion. The main themes selected are ethics: research and provision in health and social care together with service users' perspectives; followed by law, management and ethics in health and social care; with the final section on ethics: from the start of life to the end. Each chapter also sets out to identify the contemporary challenges presented for health and social care provision.

## Ethics defined

Ethics is derived from the Greek 'ethos', meaning a person's character, nature or disposition. Ethics, as relating to morals, pertains to the distinction between right and wrong or good and evil in relation to actions, volitions or the character of responsible beings. Ethical theories can cover consequentialism (assessing principles in doing good, removing harm and preventing harm) as well as virtue ethics and deontology (acting according to morally obligatory principles or duties).

Ethical principles are concerned with aspects such as: autonomy, beneficence, non-maleficence and justice; corporate, research and collaborative governance; truth telling; confidentiality; consent and accountability, the themes of which are discussed and applied across this publication. In particular, Louise Terry provides an overview of ethical principles and contemporary challenges in Chapter Two.

Each chapter addresses selected ethical principles applied to a theme in health and social care. For example, the chapter on interprofessional care (Chapter Seven) considers the issues of beneficence, confidentiality, accountability and collaborative governance in relation to interprofessional, interagency and partnership working. The purpose of this publication is to demonstrate the increasing impact of ethics on a range of themes and arenas in health and social care. The authors' chapters are summarised at the end of this introduction to provide an overview of the publication as a whole. The build-up to the rising importance of ethics is now considered in the next section on significant policy features, which shows that the place of ethics has become increasingly significant in the 21st century, which is further highlighted by the impact of the media coverage, to be illustrated shortly.

## Some significant policy features

From the beginning of the 21st century, ethics has increasingly taken a key position in publications on health and social care. In contrast, at the start of the National Health Service (NHS) from July 1948 onwards, the main focus over the postwar years concentrated on finance and provision (covering quality, quantity, access and the structural context). Over the second half of the 20th century, the structural divisions have remained between a centralised NHS and, from the mid-1970s, local authority social services covering childcare as well as care for older people, people with mental ill health, mentally handicapped and physically handicapped people. However, initially both health and social care were ultimately responsible to the Department of Health and Social Security, which changed to the Department of Health at central government level in 1988 when the responsibility for social security was undertaken separately by the newly formed Department of Social Security. Local authority social services have become increasingly responsible for nursing homes, as well as for care services, residential homes and day care services (Leathard, 2003, p 33).

Over the years an array of measures for the two separate sectors to work together across the separately administered health and social services have included: joint planning, joint approaches, joint ventures, joint working, joint commissioning, joint purchasing and joint consultative committees. Nevertheless, structural divisions remain as a challenge for the 21st century.

## Public spending and regulation

A major theme under the newly elected Conservative government in 1979 was to reduce public spending. Importance was therefore attached to the need for NHS collaboration with the private and voluntary services as well as turning to informal caring from family, friends and neighbours. As demand escalated across the private and voluntary care homes, so the need for regulation became an important issue.

## Management

A second development, from 1981 onwards, was the search for better management. The Griffiths Management Inquiry Team decided to focus largely on hospital management. The central problem diagnosed was a massive failure of clearly defined management functions. The major recommendation was to establish a commitment to general management (Griffiths Report, 1983). However, this inquiry did not extend to the provision of local authority social services.

## Partnership working

With the return of the New Labour government in 1997, after 18 years of Conservative rule, one major innovation was to introduce the theme of partnership working, especially between health and social services. One of the six key principles that underlined the changes for the new NHS was to break down organisational barriers to enable the NHS to work in partnership and to forge stronger links with local authorities (Leathard, 2000).

By 2005, various policy developments have been seeking to integrate the health and social care services, more particularly through *care trusts* (discussed in Chapter Seven); *intermediate care* that enables older people to lead more independent lives supported by health authorities, primary care groups, hospitals and local authorities, all seeking to work together; and the *2001 Health and Social Care Act* that gives the government powers to direct local authorities and health authorities to pool their budgets especially where services are failing. Nevertheless, despite these and other initiatives (Leathard, 2003, p 31) the structural divisions still remain between health and social care which therefore represent a contemporary challenge for the future.

# The rise of ethics

Meanwhile, building up to the start of the 21st century, the theme of ethics has become a major arena for consideration in publications, conferences and committees on health and social care as well as extending to wider fields. Why the position of ethics has become a central theme of interest may be explained by the wish to extend the debate and guidance on health and social care more widely to encompass the place of moral principles, codes and duties. In contrast, from 1948 to the turn of the century, the previous issues of central importance, as reviewed earlier, such as finance, service provision, reduction in public spending, management then partnership working, are all largely linked to financial and policy determinants. Rather differently, ethics introduces a more reflective, philosophical aspect while also based on clear lines of guidance where professional codes are relevant to the provision of health and social care.

## *Wider ethical developments*

From 2000 onwards, a brief review of the dates of some significant issues in ethics show how the subject has also become of increasing significance in the 21st century not only across health and social care but across wider fields as well.

- The *Royal Academy of Engineering* has recently worked with the individual engineering institutions to explore the fundamental ethical principles at the core of the engineering profession. Further, together with a range of disciplines outside engineering, such as medicine and philosophy, a high level statement of 'Ethical principles for engineers', together with a curriculum map for the teaching of ethics on undergraduate courses, has been assembled (The Royal Academy of Engineering, 2005).
- *Genetics:* rather differently, an unprecedented nationwide consultation has been launched by the Human Genetics Commission to draw out public views on new developments in genetic science, such as the screening of embryos for genetic disorders and the prospect of 'designer babies'. A discussion document outlines the perceived major issues at stake together with the associated societal and ethical implications. The responses to the report on *Choosing the future: Genetics and reproductive decision making* were to be reviewed and placed in the Commission's report to the Department of Health in late 2005 (Sample, 2005).

- *Universities:* Baroness Warwick, Chief Executive of Universities UK, has reported that universities and their staff already follow a range of codes of ethics, such as those relating to research and professional bodies. A sense of ethics and values permeates institutional approaches to staff, students and communities, from the proper conduct of staff to appropriate behaviour on campus. However, universities would welcome the opportunity to share experience with business for mutual benefit, while business representatives have called on universities to defend high moral and ethical standards (Tysome, 2004).

  In relations with students, the view that universities need to establish ethical policies is gaining ground. Universities have policies on specific areas such as ethical research but none have general ethical policies according to Richard Brown, Chief Executive of the Council for Industry and Higher Education, who has highlighted the need for every university to work out its own ethical policy before problems erupt (Macleod and Curtis, 2005).

  Meanwhile, academic pioneers at Leeds University are 'blazing a trail' by embedding ethics in all student courses in response to a growing national awareness of the need for a more explicit ethical dimension in higher education (Lipsett, 2005).

## Media coverage

From the end of the 20th century, articles, debates and publications on various aspects of ethics have increasingly become available across the arena of health and social care.

### New ethics code for BBC

In June 2005, the BBC's codes on ethics, impartiality, taste and decency have been updated. Many of the changes in the codes reflect the demands of 24-hour news and broadcasting stories on the Internet (*The Guardian*, 2005, p 10).

### Clean Investment Campaign

One interesting angle has been the Clean Investment Campaign when Roy Hemmings started to question why local health authorities, trusts and medical charities invested money in arms-exporting companies. The Campaign Against Arms Trade (CAAT) then raised the issue as to whether professions dedicated to preserving life and alleviating suffering should invest in and profit from the arms trade. The Clean Investment Campaign was then set up to persuade public bodies to avoid giving support to trading in arms (Hemmings, 1998).

## Launch of ethical investment initiative

Financial institutions that manage £1,100 billion of assets have promised to haul ethical investment into the mainstream with the launch of the Principles for Responsible Investment, crafted with the United Nations and launched at the New York Stock Exchange. The media set out six guiding principles, which comprised environmental, social and corporate issues with the aim to set up sustainable, environmental and social policies as well as the pooling of resources. However, environmental groups greeted the launch of this ethical investment initiative with scepticism (Teather, 2006).

## Socially responsible investment

By 2006, directors of groups quoted on the London Stock Exchange have been facing a new challenge: ethically or socially responsible investment. Ethical fund managers have far more power than the size of their funds would suggest as all firms are now graded, which has a significant impact on their operations in dealing with shares along ethical lines (Levene, 2006).

The above examples illustrate how ethics have become an important aspect of recent developments across a wide range of differing organisations, bodies and fields of interest.

## Medical training

Meanwhile, the British Medical Association (BMA) has hit the headlines with a call for an urgent review of ethics training in the UK as medical schools are failing to take the subject seriously even though ethics is an accepted element in medical training. The BMA has called on the government to fund a nationwide study to establish how ethics and law are taught in different institutions. The BMA has also launched a new edition of a handbook on ethics and law as the BMA believes that good ethics training is vital to enable doctors to care for patients appropriately and to deal with the increasingly complex ethical and legal dilemmas that doctors will encounter in their work. While medical ethics is an accepted element of all undergraduate courses, experts suspect that the quality and quantity of teaching vary considerably (Farrer, 2003).

## The ethical shopper

On a lighter note, Dominic Murphy assembles a weekly commentary on 'The ethical shopper' in the press. Among other examples, Murphy (2006a) has described: a range of ethical clothing selling organic t-shirts and fair trade clothing; super-efficient light bulbs that convert 90% of the energy used into light compared with 10% from the traditional equivalent (Murphy, 2006b); as well as an introduction to the launch of biomelifestyle.com which is a website dedicated to ethically sourced products for the home (Murphy, 2006c).

## Ethical energy policy

A final example of the impact of ethics comes from a very different sphere when the Conservative Party leader, David Cameron, launched his ethical energy policy by urging party members to switch their domestic electricity accounts to a renewable supplier (Kirwan-Taylor, 2006).

The above illustrations show how ethics has become a significant aspect of recent developments across a wide range of differing organisations, bodies and fields of interests. However, whatever impact ethical issues may have on the provision of health and social care, no ethical item can measure up to the fundamental importance of the current financial situation where the collective debts of the NHS had reached £1.3 billion by June 2006 (Carvel, 2006). The financial demands still remain the most significant contemporary challenge in the provision of health and social care.

## Introduction to the topic areas

This publication sets out to chart the mounting interest, widespread developments and increasing impact of ethics on health and social care alongside the contemporary challenges involved. The chapters have been assembled under the three main sections now set out.

### Section 1: Ethics: Research and provision in health and social care

Louise Terry in Chapter Two provides an introductory overview by drawing attention to the constantly evolving context of ethics that covers a wide range of theories and principles such as normative ethics, rights, consequentialism, virtue ethics, principlism, autonomy, beneficence, non-maleficence, justice and fidelity. Furthermore, the context extends to the place of ethics in law, professional codes of conduct and decision-making models. With two or more approaches to an issue, ethical dilemmas can arise. However, a series of models set out can aid health and social care professionals to move forward with procedural objectivity. The clinical and social care ethics model (Table 2.1) greatly assists towards enabling health and social care professionals to address the uni-professional perspective often brought to bear on ethical dilemmas.

In Chapter Three, Robert Stanley and Susan McLaren look at ethical issues in health and social care research. A need for the ethical regulation of research has arisen from incidents that have led to the abuse and exploitation of research participants. The recent inception of research governance frameworks in many countries is addressing the need to safeguard the rights, dignity and well-being of participants and to improve research quality through rigorous scrutiny. In the UK new and complex arrangements for ethical review, within the governance framework, have raised a number of issues that need resolution to avoid lengthy delays and increased costs of research. A need has been identified to support research ethics committees in improving quality, consistency and transparency of decision making, improving guidance, establishing clear policies and clarifying the role of ethical review, as opposed to other forms of governance scrutiny required by NHS trusts. The developing role of data monitoring committees for randomised controlled clinical trials also needs delineating from that of other review committees. In a wider context, continuing concerns exist about the participation of vulnerable groups in research and the need for continued international debate and consensus guidance to avoid the risk of exploitation.

Elaine Pierce, in Chapter Four, looks at research governance for health and social care. Governance is intended to provide a framework through which institutions are ultimately accountable for the scientific quality, moral acceptability and safety of research that meets rational, ethical, legal and research practice standards. Research governance in health and social care encompasses meeting criteria for scientific review of research proposals, ethical approval, sponsorship and supervision. Implementation of a framework should create an environment in which research can be conducted without contravening participants' moral or legal rights, by clearly delineating accountabilities of those involved, by prevention of fraud and unethical conduct. Support for implementing frameworks can be drawn from legislation, guidance and standards espoused by professional bodies and associations. In the UK, research governance frameworks state that groups representing users and carers should be involved in the research process in all or any stages.

Ethical practice includes demonstrating probity and professionalism in the use of professional status and in relationships with colleagues. The nature of general practice in the UK is changing but strong ethical principles to underpin virtuous practice are important to assure the quality of the care delivered as the patients cared for become better informed and more consumerist in their approach to health care. In Chapter Five, Charles Campion-Smith reviews the arena in the light of four ethical principles: beneficence, non-maleficence, autonomy and research governance, all of which play a significant part in general practice.

Examples of the values and ethical codes that aim to inform and govern practice are described in the overlapping domains of social care and social work in the UK. In Chapter Six, Colin and Margaret Whittington review the history and nature of three broad streams of values that influence social care and social work – 'traditional', 'emancipatory' and 'governance'. The two discussions of provenance and different value streams are included to argue that codes manifest political and organisational dimensions as well as professional ones. The authors discuss the interorganisational dimension as well as a critical context for implementing values in social work and social care through interagency relationships. The ethical themes of confidentiality, autonomy and justice, together with practical issues, are also considered in the light of carefully selected relevant case histories. The impact of interprofessional approaches has become increasingly relevant over the course of time.

Audrey Leathard, in Chapter Seven, looks at ethics and interprofessional care. The four ethical principles of beneficence, confidentiality, accountability and collaborative governance are reviewed in the light of the rising importance of collaborative governance in working together across health and social care, termed interprofessional care. Care trusts also come under focus where structurally some 32 local health and social care services have amalgamated into joint trusts. Collaborative governance is shown to have played a significant part in the context of joint provision across the services involved. However, while the term 'partnership working' has increasingly come to the fore in this context, a key ethical issue is that partnerships must ensure that the arrangements benefit users.

The place of people using the services is of major importance but requires public reassurance that the arrangements are meeting the needs of the service users appropriately. Chapter Eight, by Jill Manthorpe and Martin Stevens, has therefore considered the involvement of service users in service planning, delivery, research and evaluation. The case is argued that such involvement is both ethical as well as effective. However, a number of issues for involving service users in research and service development have been identified which include funding requirements, consultation fatigue and the increased emphasis on managerialism in public places that makes matters harder for service users to have a genuine input or control in developments.

## Section 2: Law, management and ethics in health and social care

In Chapter Nine, Louise Terry looks at the ethical and legal perspectives on human rights. Human rights legislation continues to exert an impact on health and social care through, for example, the work of the World Health Organisation. Rights legislation attempts to define parameters between interests of the individual and the state. International rights documentation encompasses that of legally binding countries that have ratified conventions and that which relates to guidelines incorporated into the declarations of international bodies. Vulnerable groups (for example, children, older people, disabled pregnant women, those with mental illness) are singled out for special protection in many conventions. In the UK, health and social care organisations, subject to the 1998 Human Rights Act, must consider service users' rights balancing individual and community interests; increasingly courts are involved in decision making arising from the assertion of rights. Many individuals, groups and populations have limited access to health and social care services and cannot sustain their rights: a continuing challenge for the international community.

Robert Irvine and John McPhee, in Chapter Ten, look at Australian perspectives on multidisciplinary team practice in law and ethics. Collaborative teamwork in health care settings tends to be an indeterminate, multifaceted social and moral idea. As a result, teamwork covers a range of different practices, ideologies and institutions. Through the analogy of the 'captain of the ship', the success of teamwork is shown to depend on strategies for governing complex assemblies of individual conduct, collective action, technologies, space and communication. The relationship between ethics and multidisciplinary teamwork reflects the fact that not all aspects of teamwork are or must be ethical, but the arena is morally relevant. What matters ethically is seen to be how professionals respond to others whose difference is recognised so that the actual participation in interdisciplinary dialogue is extended and cultivated. The process of making, maintaining and reproducing teams requires a system of ethics capable of responding effectively and productively to ethical thought and action that can be applied in a combination of different contexts.

In Chapter Eleven, Jeff Girling looks at ethics and the management of health and social care. Also considered is the place of responding to ethical situations through intuition, values, rules and codes, principles and theory as well as action. In thinking ethically and working practically, developments have led to a growth of top-down targets, inspection and audit regimes, bidding processes for funding sources and numerous plans and strategies. Managers are faced with choice. There is plenty of choice for freedom at the organisational level in the health and social care services where developments also include system working, joint planning and partnership arrangements, clinical networks, new types of organisations such as foundation trusts and independent sector models. As a manager in health and social care, a sense of justice and of caring are both needed in order to be concerned about organisational performance and viability, about eliminating waste and about meeting needs. The ethical dimension can fit uncomfortably with other managerial attributes such as hiring and firing, setting up quality assurance systems, making firm decisions and managing change.

Mary Dombeck and Tobie Hittle Olsan, in Chapter Twelve, look at a US perspective on ethics and the social responsibility of institutions regarding resource allocation in health and social care. In the US the context of health care is defined by the ability of the service users to pay for services through insurance and by the availability of service provision. Unemployed people are therefore especially vulnerable to being uninsured. The health care system is therefore complex with disparate care and services for different populations that place ethical burdens on the providers. However, evidence has shown from the behaviour of health care consumers that patients value provider–patient relationships. The ethical challenge, linked to the theme of justice, therefore remains to prevent the loss of morally responsible personhood in institutions by enhancing the connection of people to their institutions so that socially responsible decisions can be made.

In Chapter Thirteen, Bridget Penhale looks at ethics and charging for care. In the UK an increased emphasis has been placed on charging for social care that has engendered debate relating to the extent to which older people should pay for care needs and the scope of provision in publicly funded care. Inconsistency exists in the national financing of long-term care provision. In Scotland, free personal care is available; in England, Wales and Northern Ireland free nursing care in care homes is available but not free personal care. Care managers can encounter conflicts in personal care and professional values, leading to ethical dilemmas, for example in the areas of financial assessment, services, deprivation of assets and charging for services. Issues arising in relation to fairness and administrative justice include variations in policies, practices and procedures between authorities and the need for consistency; variations in levels of charges and means of calculation for social services raise issues for equity. Practices in charging for care could be improved through provision of training for managers and professionals in ethics and financial assessment; the development of improved transparent systems of support and supervision; and better communication and information exchange between professionals, users and carers.

## Section 3: Ethics: From the start of life to the end

Brenda Almond, in Chapter Fourteen, looks at ethical challenges and the new technologies of reproduction. Advances in genetics, together with developments and applications in new reproductive technologies, raise a number of challenging questions, not least of which is the extent to which the law should control developments. Through new technologies, children can be born to individuals to whom they are not related. Such children may not have wider family networks, relationships and a related sense of identity, raising questions about the concept of family as a social, legal and biological construct. International consensus on human rights defends the freedom of two individuals to marry and have children and also the possibility of bringing children into the world who are not genetically related to individuals who are from their circle or network. In deploying new technologies, society has a responsibility to perfect the rights of people at a vulnerable stage of their development when, as such, they cannot be protected. Rights about genetic relatives, knowledge of origins, future roles and choices need to be considered. In some countries, legislation has been enacted that establishes a right for individuals born via gamete donation to know the identity of their genetic parent. Risks exist that could jeopardise the principle of the equal dignity of individuals and lead to a failure to protect people with negative consequences.

In Chapter Fifteen, David Hodgson looks at ethics and caring for children and young people. The starting point for considering valuations of children alongside professional discretion is discussed in the light of the government Green Paper *Every child matters* (DfES, 2003), which contained proposals to reform children's services following the report into Victoria Climbié's death. Several of the proposals resulted in legal changes introduced in the 2004 Children Act. Relationships, interests and rights have been reviewed in the light of the moral debates regarding the care of children from which a reformulation of the link between rights and discretion is suggested. Several pathways are set out to promote human rights in childcare practice: personal integrity and the definitions of abuse; the representation of children's voices; safeguarding children through family support; and personal and professional competence. A conceptual and historical analysis of childcare discourse has helped to identify ethical challenges in the form of several pathways for the pursuit of professional justice and respect for human rights: advocating children's equal rights to physical and emotional integrity; recognising personal privacy as central to child protection; maximising formal and informal structures to represent the perspectives of young people; using skill and judgement to further models of competence building with children, families and professionals; and, finally, addressing the contradictions in law and policy that encourage judgemental attitudes, undermine professional creativity and detract from family support. All elements need to be brought together to operate effectively.

In Chapter Sixteen, Keith Andrews looks at ethical dilemmas in caring for people with complex disabilities. Complex disabilities can result in a diverse range and combination of physical, cognitive and behavioural disorders that can impact variably on the individual, family and society. Ethical decision making is informed by the principles of respect for autonomy, beneficence, non-maleficence and justice. Dilemmas can arise in relation to decision making for those who lack mental capacity, withholding or withdrawing treatment, confidentiality and involvement in teaching and publication. Where mental capacity is lacking, decisions must be in the best interests of the people and the least restrictive option chosen that balances duty of care with personal freedom. 'Best interest' requires net benefits and possible futility of treatment to be considered. In weighing benefits and possible burdens of treatment, doctors cannot substitute their own values or focus solely on the benefits of treatment; consideration must be given to what a person's wishes would have been. Challenges inherent in acting in best interests are the risks of imposing the values of the able-bodied.

Jon Glasby, Helen Lester and Emily McKie, in Chapter Seventeen, look at the area of mental health. The proposed changes to the 1983

Mental Health Act are considered to focus on risk and public safety rather than on the health and welfare of those people whose decision making is impaired through their mental disorder. The authors also consider that the draft Mental Health Bill (2004) is not in keeping with other current relevant government policy initiatives, particularly the choice agenda. The outcome could disadvantage people with mental health problems relative to other patients' groups. The currently proposed legislation would appear to be limited to this group because resources tend to be limited to the increasing number of people under compulsion. A better way forward for risk reduction is the suggestion that patients should be encouraged to feel able to seek help early on, to be encouraged to talk about their fears and problems, then become involved, where needed, with accessible, effective, responsive and appropriate services. At the centre of the ethical dilemma in this field is the need to balance the rights of the individual with mental illness and the welfare and safety of the wider public.

In Chapter Eighteen, Anthea Tinker looks at ethics and older people. General and demographic factors are examined to assess the ethical case for and against treating older people differently from other age groups. The argument for treating older people as a special group is the perception that this age group is more likely to be physically and mentally disabled; but there are arguments for and against this viewpoint. Points are then set out surrounding the ethical issues in the provision of health and social care to older people that cover questions such as: should treatment and care be given on the basis of need? Are there circumstances in which the age of the person should be taken into account and, if so, what are the relevant issues? Older people are also more likely to receive a higher proportion of health and social care services than their proportion of the population would justify. At this point, the place of ethics is shown to be relevant regarding the question of age discrimination. As the number of older people in society increases annually and is set to escalate proportionately ever more across the 21st century, the place of older people and how their needs are to be met will probably set one of the most challenging ethical and financial problems for the future, alongside the key issues discussed in this chapter on consent, autonomy and confidentiality. Of all the chapters in this publication, ethics and older people will become an ever-increasing challenge to society — financially, ethically and morally.

In Chapter Nineteen, Clive Seale looks at ethics and euthanasia. The arena is problematical. Public support for laws that allow medical practitioners to end life by active measures in the UK has risen but the medical profession has shown reluctance to endorse the practice of euthanasia. Surveys of the relatives and friends of people who have died as well as surveys on medical practitioners involved in euthanasia are reviewed to illustrate the moral and ethical dilemmas in this field. Studies by the author and colleagues on, for example, the role of hospice and palliative care show just how complex and sensitive this field of care is, which presents constant challenges such as the balance to be achieved between the continuing importance of the avoidance of harms while attempting to ensure that a system does not deny benefits to a small proportion of people who would otherwise endure much suffering. A further contemporary challenge exists, particularly in the field of work where valuable discussion is set out on international comparisons. So one contemporary challenge in this field remains. Why and how can one country in Europe – such as the Netherlands – have access to a form of medical help that is denied to other European countries, for what are perceived as very ethical grounds? The question underlines a key challenge for the 21st century in a field of deeply held personal and professional views.

Across this publication, the central theme of ethics is applied to a wide range of front-runner issues in health and social care in the UK and abroad. The three main sections cover the key elements of research and provision, law and management, with the final emphasis on looking at the implications of ethics across the varying life stages. Above all, the contemporary challenges are highlighted throughout.

## References

Carvel, J. (2006) 'Cutbacks threat as NHS deficits hit £1.3bn', *The Guardian*, 8 June, p 6.

DfES (Department for Education and Skills) (2003) *Every child matters: Summary*, London: The Stationery Office.

Farrer, S. (2003) 'Call for urgent review of UK ethics training', *The Times Higher*, 19 May, p 12.

Griffiths Report (1983) *NHS management inquiry*, London: DHSS.

*Guardian, The* (2004) 'FTSE sets up ethics indices', 15 December, p 21.

*Guardian, The* (2005) 'New ethics code for BBC', 23 June, p 5.

Hemmings, R. (1998) 'Into the arms of the NHS', *Health Matters*, issue 31, pp 12-13.

Kirwan-Taylor, H. (2006) 'David Cameron has launched his ethical energy policy', *The Evening Standard*, 18 January, pp 20-1.

Leathard, A. (2000) *Health care provision: Past, present and into the 21st century* (2nd edn), Cheltenham: Stanley Thornes (Publishers) Ltd.

Leathard, A. (2003) *Interprofessional collaboration from policy to practice in health and social care*, London: Brunner-Routledge.

Levene, T. (2006) 'Your money in their hands', *The Guardian*, 22 April, p 4.

Lipsett, A. (2005) 'Pioneers set ethics at heart of courses', *The Times Higher*, 30 September, p 56.

Macleod, D. and Curtis, P. (2005) 'Whose line is it anyway?', *Education Guardian*, 4 October, p 12.

Murphy, D. (2006a) 'The ethical shopper' (on clothing), *The Guardian*, 7 March, p 27.

Murphy, D. (2006b) 'The ethical shopper: seeing the light', *The Guardian*, 18 April, p 23.

Murphy, D. (2006c) 'The ethical shopper' (on ethical products for the home), *The Guardian*, 14 February, p 7.

Royal Academy of Engineering, The (2005) *Ethics and the engineer: Embedding ethics in the engineering community*, London: Royal Academy of Engineering.

Sample, I. (2004) 'National consultation on designer babies', *The Guardian*, 16 July, p 9.

Teather, D. (2006) 'Scepticism greets launch of ethical investment initiative', *The Guardian*, 28 April, p 31.

Tysome, T. (2004) 'Uphold morals, industry tells v–cs', *The Times Higher*, 11 June, p 10.

# Section 1
## Ethics: Research and provision in health and social care

# TWO

# Ethics and contemporary challenges in health and social care

*Louise Terry*

## Summary

This chapter briefly explains ethical theories, principles and issues of relevance in health and social care including some recent trends in contemporary policy and practice with ethical implications. The first section, 'What is "ethics"?', separates ethics from morality. The question 'What is "ethics"?' leads to an examination of distinctions between normative and non-normative ethics, virtue ethics, ethics and law. In 'Applied and professional ethics', examples of ethical challenges are identified highlighting issues common to health and social care. Finally, the changing nature of professional roles and relationships, the role of protocols in relation to professional autonomy, lack of trust, changing social trends, potentially infinite demand with finite resources, increasing ethnic diversity, policy drivers towards quality and targets and a focus on risk assessment and risk management are explored.

## What is 'ethics'?

'Ethics' and 'morals' are often used interchangeably. A useful separation is to use 'morals' for those personal values and beliefs formulated in the uniqueness of our individual life experiences and 'ethics' in relation to professional values and philosophies. Beauchamp and Childress (2001) argue that philosophical ethics form the highest level of abstraction from which key principles can be extracted. These principles may then be reshaped as rules guiding behaviours. Professional ethics can be defined as the philosophy or principles central to the accepted attitudes and behaviours of a professional group such as nurses, doctors or social workers. Most professional groups articulate the rights and responsibilities of their members via rules or codes of professional conduct, the breaching of which may result in censure or exclusion from the professional group, since ethical decision making cannot rest solely on individual moral judgement. The word 'ethics' is derived from 'ethos', Greek for character or disposition. Health and social care professionals are expected to demonstrate certain characteristics such as caring, empathy, honesty and trustworthiness.

## Ethical theory and principles

Falling into a trap of believing that "cultures manifest preferences, motivations and evaluations so wide and chaotic in their variety that no values nor practical principles can be said to be evident to human beings" is easy as these issues are so wide, and "no value or practical principle is recognised in all times and all places..." (Finnis, 1980, p 83). Ethical theory is constantly evolving from the virtue ethics espoused 2,500 years ago to the Rights movements and Gaian (environmentalist) ethics of the 20th century. The philosophical focus may be on the individual or on society. This next section briefly outlines key philosophies.

### Normative ethics

Normative theories of ethics rely on a notion of doing what ought to be done and tend to be rule-based. Deontology ('deon' is Greek for duty) represents one of the oldest moral philosophies. Judaism, Christianity and Islam have key rules or duties (for example, 'thou shalt not kill') that should be obeyed by adherents. Immanuel Kant (1724–1804) developed a duty-based ethics that focuses on the practical reasoning skills and goodwill of the actor rather than divine rules. Rational human intelligence is used to discover what is right. Actions are moral if the actor has goodwill. In other words, the actor does what he ought to do while recognising that this is what ought to be done, not because the consequences will be good.

Respecting others as moral agents is central, for example, gaining consent to medical treatment and involving people with disabilities in the design of home support interventions. People should never be used for the benefit of another or society: "Treat humanity whether in thine own person or in that of any other, in every case as an end withal, never as a means to an end" (Kant, 1724–1804, p 38). For instance, when respecting the 'Golden Rule' ('do unto others as you would have them do unto you'), a test of whether this action should *always* be taken should be applied. If a community psychiatric nurse were asked by a patient who has threatened his ex-wife where she lives, Kantian ethics suggests that lying about her whereabouts is wrong because allowing lying shows disrespect and erodes trust. That one ought always to tell the truth is a 'categorical imperative' no matter how hard or how unpleasant the consequences might be. This 'categorical imperative' is expressed as: "I ought never to act otherwise than so that I could also will that my maxim should become a universal law" (Kant, 1724-1804, p 15). Professional codes of conduct are usually deontologically based but duties may conflict and a dilemma arises.

## Rights

One of the earliest statements of human rights is the English *Magna Carta* (1215), which includes the right not to be imprisoned without fair trial. In the case of *R v Bournewood Mental Health Trust, ex parte L* [1999] AC 458, a man with severe autism was detained in a psychiatric hospital as a 'voluntary' patient. Although his 'detention' was eventually held lawful, the lack of protection for vulnerable people was strongly criticised.

Rights are extremely powerful (Dworkin, 1977). A legal right not to be discriminated against can only be ignored in limited circumstances. The concept is one of 'liberal individualism': within a democratic society, individuals have protected rights and freedoms (Beauchamp and Childress, 2001, p 70). International declarations on human rights and national constitutions set standards regarding relationships between states and citizens. Sub-sets of rights (feminist, gay, black etc) advance the status and freedoms of minority groups. However, often one person's 'rights' conflict with another's. Patients with equal rights to treatment compete for hospital beds. In social work, a child's rights might be pitted against their parents'. Some see rights as absolute and unchallengeable. Nozick (1974, p 74) asserts: "Individuals have rights and there are things that no person or group can do to them", but without a notion of reciprocal responsibilities, anarchy arises. In reality, some rights are seen as 'concrete' (having firm foundations in laws like the 1995 Disability Discrimination Act); other rights are seen more as aspirations, such as 'the right to the highest attainable standard of physical and mental health'.

## Consequentialism

Consequentialists believe the morality of an action depends on the balance of its consequences. The best-known version is utilitarianism. Jeremy Bentham (1748-1832, pp 12-13) wrote: "An action may ... be said to be conformable to the principle of utility ... when ... the tendency which it has to augment the happiness of the community is greater than any which it has to diminish it". The end justifies the means. Difficulty arises in deciding what is the good of the community or whose 'happiness' counts. Are all consequences foreseeable? John Stuart Mill (1806-73) developed a concept of utilitarianism that saw human flourishing ('eudaemonia') as key. Decisions should be made according to how they further human welfare.

Other problems arise in that strict ('Act') utilitarianism focuses solely on the act in question. Sacrificing one healthy individual to provide life-saving transplants for several others becomes acceptable. Unless specific protections are incorporated individual rights become meaningless. Therefore, 'Rule' utilitarianism incorporates rules such as not killing although encouragement of an ethos that older people have fewer rights to life-saving treatment than the young is allowable. Much public policy is utilitarian (Beauchamp and Childress, 2001, p 55). Resource allocation in health and social care often focuses on achieving 'the greatest good for the greatest number'. Singer (1993), a modern utilitarian, distinguishes preventing harm from promoting good, as there is a greater obligation to do the former. Service pressures may cause harm as, for example, when patients with mental ill health remain in the community potentially at risk to themselves or others (Cooling, 2002). Although consequentialist theories are often portrayed as opposite to normative ones, in real life there is a blurring between theories and between theory and action.

## Communitarianism and social contractarianism

Under communitarianism, decisions are grounded on a concept of mutuality of obligations within the community. Marxism represents a militant form in contrast to gentler versions such as the devolvement of decision making to local groups such as primary care groups (a current British example).

Social contractarians argue that there is a moral 'contract' between the governed and the governing. The governed pay their taxes, obey the law and, in return, the government or ruler looks after their interests.

Rawls (1972) posits that the social contract requires systems maximising liberty and minimising difference (inequality) between individuals.

## Virtue ethics

Virtue ethics focus on the character of the actor. Courage, integrity, generosity and compassion are some of the traits to which to aspire. People possessing the virtues will do 'right' (Aristotle, 384–322 BC). Catholic, Jewish and Islamic medical ethics are strongly grounded in virtue ethics. A secular, virtue-based ethics seems appropriate in the health and social care professions because the work involves caring relationships (Rhodes, 1986). Health and social care professionals are commonly accepted as having certain values inculcated in them through training and socialisation that will guide their future decision making but the ad hoc nature of moral/ethical training makes this problematic.

## Principlism

Beauchamp and Childress (2001) argue powerfully in favour of a principle-based approach to ethics. The principles of autonomy (self-governance), beneficence (providing benefit), non-maleficence (avoiding harm) and justice (fairness) are seen as central to the complex relationships between patients, clients, families and the people and organisations providing care (O'Neill, 2002, p 124). These principles are supported by rules regarding confidentiality, veracity (truth telling) and privacy (Beauchamp and Childress, 2001).

## Autonomy

Autonomy has become increasingly important, partly through a stronger focus on rights, which is often reflected in legislation and case law supporting patient/client choice. At its simplest, autonomy means a right to choose, or refuse, care. Tension can arise between liberal traditions embracing a strong sense of autonomy and more communitarian cultures. Family values may be ignored as irrelevant. Autonomy may, however, be supported inappropriately. For example, patients with mental ill health with paranoid delusions have been deemed autonomous enough to refuse treatment for life-threatening physical illnesses (Terry, 2003). Aglich (2003, p 178) argues that "full autonomy implies the possession of capacities that form the apex of a broad and tall pyramid" and ethicists have oversimplified the "complex reality of disability and dependence". In Europe, a more paternalistic approach may still be seen as appropriate (Surbone et al, 2004).

## Beneficence, non-maleficence and justice

The principles of beneficence and non-maleficence are frequently seen as two sides of the same coin. However, while a positive obligation not to harm exists, providing benefit is not always possible. Diseases may be incurable, disability irreversible. Sometimes choices have to be made between patients or clients – not everyone will receive as much care as needed. The principle of justice is one of the hardest to apply. Fairness is required in the allocation of resources such as money, time, beds and drugs. Governments and care organisations worldwide struggle to balance limited resources against individual demand (NACCHDSS, 1993; Blumstein, 1997; Romanoff, 2002; Wanless, 2002). Sometimes only procedural fairness results leaving those in need and their families feeling betrayed.

## Fidelity

Ultimately, the principle of fidelity (keeping faith) is vital. Health and social care practitioners have to keep faith:

- with the patient or client by avoiding harm and respecting, supporting and enhancing autonomy, however residual, or carefully weighing benefits and burdens, knowing what to take into account, when the recipient of care is unable to act autonomously;
- with their profession by observing their code of conduct;
- with their employer by meeting organisational goals and standards, including the need for interprofessional working;
- with society by adhering to national policy frameworks, meeting legal standards and by obeying the law;
- with themselves – maintaining personal integrity is important.

Tensions arise between different principles and between principles and practice (Wall, 2003, p 71). Developing critical self-reflection skills helps improve ethical behaviours and working practices (Leppa and Terry, 2004).

## Ethics and law

Not every moral obligation has a corresponding legal duty. Not every law is moral. Whether law need be moral is debatable. However comforting the belief that "every legal duty is founded on a moral obligation" (*R v Instan* [1893] 1 QB 453), arguably, as long as the law has been made in accordance with correct procedures, by a body with requisite legislative powers, the moral content is irrelevant. Some argue that, as moral agents, people should disobey 'immoral' laws, regardless of the personal consequences (the 'Nazi' law defence). Doctors have carried out euthanasia regardless of the law.

Legal decision making relies on rules regarding the interpretation of statutes and decisions in earlier cases. Judges are trained in law not ethics. In cases involving children, the English judiciary's freedom to consider the welfare of siblings is severely restricted under current legislation. What might be best for one child might be devastating for a sibling. In jurisdictions allied to England, an adversarial approach is taken which means that, when resorted to in complex medical and social care cases, the search for 'truth' or 'morally right action' (which European courts are more likely to do as part of their inquisitorial approach) is hindered.

## Applied and professional ethics

### Professional codes of conduct

Health and social care practitioners and managers are expected to obey their professional codes of conduct or have the right to practice removed. Respecting patient/client autonomy, beneficence, non-maleficence and confidentiality are common deontological features. Codification of ethics is problematic, however, due to the lack of commonality (Seedhouse, 2002). Priorities may differ between professions. Tackling suspected abuse of children or older people is one area where health and social care professionals might struggle to reach concord. When each profession faces excessive workloads and inadequate resources, mistakes may be made as in the Climbié case (Secretary of State for Health and Secretary of State for the Home Department, 2003). Sometimes, individuals act in a way they believe is required only to be punished (BBC News, 2005a). A small knowledge of ethical theory and membership of a profession is little help in resolving complex ethical decisions.

## Decision-making models

An ethical dilemma exists when there are two or more possible approaches to a situation. A number of models exist to assist decision makers but they rarely give a definitive, absolute answer to an ethical dilemma. Their usefulness is in helping health and social care professionals explore relevant aspects and demonstrate procedural objectivity. The least helpful approach is to accept uncritically that what is ethical varies from situation to situation.

Jonsen et al's (1998) clinical ethics model can be adapted to fit both health and social care. The model in Table 2.1 helps extract and record all information that might impact on the decision. How that information is balanced is then a matter of judgement.

This modified model can be used by health and social care professionals to help address the uni-professional perspective that, too often, is brought to bear on ethical dilemmas. An example of a challenging ethical dilemma involving health and social care professionals is that of planning the discharge from hospital of a patient who would prefer to return home but the home environment has been assessed as unsuitable. The modified Jonsen model enables a balanced approach to be taken. Information relevant to health and social care needs as well as patient preferences and other contextual issues can be extracted.

An alternative approach is to apply the Beauchamp and Childress (2001) principles of autonomy, beneficence, non-maleficence and justice to ethical dilemmas along with other relevant principles and rules such as fidelity and confidentiality. In the example of patient discharge from hospital, the principle of autonomy requires that the patient's wishes be heard. However, the principles of beneficence and non-maleficence may suggest that patient safety has to be prioritised over autonomy if the patient's autonomy is impaired. The principle of justice in fairness of allocation of resources suggests that a timely discharge from hospital is needed. Justice also suggests that patients with the financial resources to contribute to the costs of social care should do so. Resolution of such ethical dilemmas sometimes requires decisions to be made that are not in the best interests of all parties. For example, relatives take on the burden of care at the expense of their own welfare. The principle of fidelity requires honesty with the patient and others over the available options and costs.

Ward managers in a hospital may face conflict between professional nursing values and the often-utilitarian nature of service delivery. Professional nursing values may suggest that a patient's discharge is

**Table 2.1:** Clinical and social care ethics model

| Medical and Social Care Indicators | Personal preferences |
|---|---|
| 1. What is the person's: medical problem? history? diagnosis? prognosis? | 1. What has the person expressed about preferences for treatment? |
| 2. Is the medical problem: acute? chronic? critical? emergent? reversible? | 2 Has s/he been informed about benefits and risks, understood and given consent? |
| 3. What are the person's social care problems? infirmity? paralysis? learning difficulties? mental illness? dementia? | 3. What has the person expressed about preferences for social care? |
| 4. Are the social care problems: acute? chronic? critical? emergent? reversible? | 4. Has s/he been informed about benefits and costs, understood and given consent? |
| 5. How do the social care problems and medical problems interact? Is a risk posed to others? | 5. Is the person mentally capable and legally competent? What evidence is there of incapacity? |
| 6. What are the goals of treatment and care? | 6. Has the person expressed prior preferences eg advance directive regarding medical treatment or a wish for a particular nursing or care home? |
| 7. What are the probabilities of successfully meeting those goals? | 7. If incapacitated, who is the appropriate surrogate decision-maker? Does this person have legal power to make both medical and financial decisions? Are appropriate standards of decision-making being employed? |
| 8. What plans exist in the case of therapeutic failure? | 8. Is the person unwilling or unable to comply with the recommended health or social care interventions? If so, why? |
| 9. In sum, how can this person be benefited by health and social care interventions and how can harm be avoided? | 9. In sum, is the person's right to choose the medical and social care they receive being respected to the extent possible in ethics and law? |

*contd.../*

*Source:* Adapted from A. Jonsen, M. Siegler and W. Winslade (1998) *Clinical Ethics* (4th edn), New York: McGraw Hill. Reproduced with permission of The McGraw Hill Company, The author is grateful to Albert Jonsen for kindly allowing his model to be adapted for the purposes of this chapter.

**Table 2.1:** contd.../

| Quality of life | Contextual features |
|---|---|
| 1. What are the prospects, with or without treatment or social care, for a return to the person's normal quality of life? | 1. Are there family issues that might influence health or social care decisions? |
| 2. Are there biases that might prejudice the provider's evaluation of that person's quality of life? | 2. Are there provider (physicians, nurses, allied health professional, social care team) issues that might influence treatment or care decisions? |
| 3. What physical, mental and social deficits is the person likely to experience if medical treatment succeeds? | 3. Are there financial and economic factors? |
| 4. Is the person's present or future condition such that continued life might be judged unacceptable by him/her? | 4. Are there religious or cultural factors? |
| 5. What plans or rationale exist to forgo treatment? | 5. Is there any justification to breach confidentiality? |
| 6. What plans or rationale exist to limit or withhold social care? | 6. Are there problems of allocations of resources? |
| 7. What plans exist for comfort and palliative care? | 7. What are the legal implications of treatment or social care decisions? |
| | 8. Is clinical research or teaching involved? |
| | 9. Are there any provider or institutional conflicts of interest? |

premature but the hospital needs to free the bed for someone else. Utilitarianism accepts that using others, such as relatives, to provide care may be best for society. In contrast, challenges to health or social care decisions may come from 'service users' or relatives arguing that they have 'rights' (Ham and McIlver, 2000). A right to a hospital or nursing home bed or social care cannot exist to the exclusion of the rights of others. The communitarian nature of state-funded health and social care delivery suggests an obligation for all parties to consider the needs of others.

## Ethical challenges in health and social care

### Changing nature of professional roles and relationships

Worldwide, health and social care professionals are widening their remits leading to a blurring of roles. Greater professional autonomy is sought despite the accompanying increase in personal accountability. Links between health, social care and other agencies involved with vulnerable people such as education and the police are being strengthened, particularly in the UK (DH, 1999; Stewart et al, 2003). Conflict often results (Cott, 1997; Malin et al, 2002, pp 100-3). Irvine (2002, p 205) notes "... each profession may define and/or explain any situation in qualitatively different ways". Lack of trust in others' expertise is evident (Hunter, 2000).

Lack of trust in professions is also evident in the rise of protocols governing behaviour and restricting professional autonomy. Many of these protocols are government responses to diminishing public trust as part of an agenda to replace "traditional relations of trust, now grown problematic, with stronger systems for securing trustworthiness" (O'Neill, 2002, p 130). Since professional status no longer automatically engenders trust (O'Neill, 2002, p 139), users of health and social services, as well as practitioners, need to work out for themselves who to trust.

### Demographic changes and public policy responses

Priority setting is one of the greatest international challenges in health and social care (Ham and Robert, 2003). Finite resources face infinite demand. Advances in medical science, leading to aging populations and more people surviving illness or accident with disabilities, coupled with higher public expectations, increase demand for care, but diminishing numbers of workers to deliver that care, funded though their taxes, means that policy makers are, therefore, seeking solutions that are fiscally, politically and legally acceptable and arguably ethical. Ham and Robert (2003) note that a focus on evidence-based medicine and cost–utility approaches characterised initial priority setting approaches in countries like the UK, Canada, New Zealand and the Netherlands with an emphasis on improving quality of care and meeting targets. More recently, the priority-setting focus has begun to recognise the importance of values (Ham and Robert, 2003, p 141). However, limited rights of appeal against resource allocation decisions, coupled with recognition that reducing risk may be uneconomical, given limits on health and social care funding, suggest that the needs of the individual will always be seen as less than those of the community.

Careers in health and social care appear less attractive to school leavers who often command higher wages elsewhere. The burden of care still traditionally falls on women (many of whom are unpaid, untrained carers of family members) and, more recently, on immigrant workers whose skills may be desperately needed in their homelands. Increasing ethnic diversity produces further challenges in responding to health or social problems unique to individual ethnic groups. The main social trends affecting care and family policies according to Malin et al (2002, p 111) are:

- geographical movement
- labour market changes
- fertility and reproduction
- changes in patterns of death, disease and disability
- changes in family formations and partnerships.

Policy makers respond with initiatives such as family-friendly working practices in the UK to encourage recruitment and retention of health and social care workers. However, maintaining staff morale is problematic. Increasing litigation has necessarily promoted the role of risk assessment, risk management and raised awareness of personal and professional liability. Tension is evident whereby pressure to meet government-set targets, such as time in Accident and Emergency departments, impacts on professional judgement. Government initiatives to increase university places have resulted in large numbers of unemployed healthcare professionals (BBC News, 2005b).

## Conclusions

Health and social care often appear characterised by each of the parties involved having differing interpretations of their roles and responsibilities as well as differing notions of what is ethically appropriate. While an understanding of ethical theory and principles helps inform debate, agreement regarding the appropriate balancing of ethics and interests is sometimes impossible to reach leaving one or more of the parties dissatisfied. Transparency regarding decision making and underpinning ethical reasoning coupled with demonstrating respect for the opinions of others is central to professional conduct. Working in health or social care has never been more challenging but, for the ethically aware professional, the arena is highly rewarding.

## References

Aglich, G. (2003) *Dependence and autonomy in old age*, Cambridge: Cambridge University Press.

Aristotle (384–322 BC) *The Nichomachean ethics*, translated by David Ross (1925) Oxford: Oxford University Press.

BBC News (2005a) 'Clark doctor guilty of misconduct', 6 August (available at http://news.bbc.co.uk).

BBC News (2005b) 'Unemployed doctors', 9 August (available at http://news.bbc.co.uk).

Beauchamp, T. and Childress, J. (2001) *Principles of biomedical ethics* (5th edn), Oxford: Oxford University Press.

Bentham, J. (1748–1832) *An introduction to the principles of morals and legislation*, an authoritative edition by J.H. Burns and H.L.A. Hart (1996) Oxford: Clarendon Press.

Blumstein, J. (1997) 'The Oregon experiment: the role of cost-benefit analysis in the allocation of Medicaid funds', *Social Science Medicine*, vol 45, no 4, pp 545-54.

Cooling, N. (2002) 'Lessons to be learnt from the Christopher Clunis story: a mental health perspective', *Clinical Risk*, vol 8, no 2, pp 52-55.

Cott, C. (1997) 'We decide, you carry it out: a social network analysis of multidisciplinary long term care teams', *Social Science and Medicine*, vol 45, no 9, pp 1411-21.

DH (Department of Health) (1999) *Saving lives: Our healthier nation*, London: The Stationery Office.

Dworkin, R. (1977) *Taking rights seriously*, Cambridge, MA: Harvard University Press.

Finnis, J. (1980) *Natural law and natural rights*, Oxford: Oxford University Press.

Ham, C. and McIlver, S. (2000) *Contested decisions: Priority setting in the NHS*, London: King's Fund Publishing.

Ham, C. and Robert, G. (2003) *Reasonable rationing: International experience of priority setting in health care*, Buckingham: Open University Press.

Hunter, D. (2000) 'Pitfalls of arranged marriages', *Health Service Journal*, vol 110, no 5729, 23 November, pp 22-3.

Irvine, R., Kerridge, I., McPhee, J. and Freeman, S. (2002) 'Interprofessionalism and ethics: consensus or clash of culture', *Journal of Interprofessional Care*, vol 16, no 3, pp 199-210.

Jonsen, A., Siegler, M. and Winslade, W. (1998) *Clinical ethics* (4th edn), New York: McGraw Hill.

Kant, I. (1724-1804) *Groundwork of the metaphysics of morals*, translated and edited by M. Gregor (1998) Cambridge: Cambridge University Press.

Leppa, C. and Terry, L. (2004) 'Reflective practice in nurse ethics education: international collaboration', *Journal of Advanced Nursing*, vol 48, no 2, pp 195-202.

Malin, N., Wilmot, S. and Manthorpe, J. (2002) *Key concepts and debates in health and social policy*, Buckingham: Open University Press.

Mill, J.S. (1806-1873) *On liberty*, edited by G. Himmelfarb (1982) Harmondsworth: Penguin.

NACCHDSS (National Advisory Committee on Core Health and Disability Support Services) (1993) *Consensus development conference report to the National Advisory Committee on Core Health and Disability Services*, Wellington, New Zealand: NACCHDSS.

Nozick, R. (1974) *Anarchy, state and utopia*, New York, NY: Basic Books.

O'Neill, O. (2002) *Autonomy and trust in bioethics*, Cambridge: Cambridge University Press.

Rawls, J. (1972) *A theory of justice*, Oxford: Oxford University Press.

Rhodes, M. (1986) *Ethical dilemmas in social work*, London: Routledge and Kegan Paul.

Romanoff, R. (2002) *Final report: Building on values: The future of health care in Canada*, Saskatchewan, Canada: CFHCC (Commission on the Future of Health Care in Canada).

Secretary of State for Health and Secretary of State for the Home Department (2003) *The Victoria Climbié Inquiry: Report of an inquiry*, London: The Stationery Office (available at www.victoria-climbie-inquiry.org.uk/).

Seedhouse, D. (2002) 'Commitment to health: a shared ethical bond between professions', *Journal of Interprofessional Care*, vol 16, no 3, pp 249-59.

Singer, P. (1993) *Practical ethics* (2nd edn), Cambridge: Cambridge University Press.

Stewart, A., Petch, A. and Curtice, L. (2003) 'Moving towards integrated working in health and social care in Scotland: from maze to matrix', *Journal of Interprofessional Care*, vol 17, no 4, pp 335-50.

Surbone, A., Ritossa, C. and Spagnolo, A.G. (2004) 'Evolution of truth-telling attitudes and practices in Italy', *Critical Reviews in Oncology/Hematology*, vol 3, pp 165-72.

Terry, L. (2003) 'The nurse's role and the NMC code of professional practice in the use of section 58 powers', *Mental Health Practice*, vol 7, no 3, pp 22-5.

Wall, A. (2003) 'Some ethical issues arising from interprofessional working', in A. Leathard (ed) *Interprofessional collaboration: From policy to practice in health and social care*, Hove: Brunner-Routledge, pp 69-78.

Wanless, D. (2002) *Securing our future health: Taking a long-term view. The final report* (available at www.hm-treasury.gov.uk/wanless).

# THREE

# Ethical issues in health and social care research

*Robert Stanley and Susan McLaren*

## Summary

Historically, research has been tainted by incidents of unethical conduct in which vulnerable individuals were harmed. This chapter reviews events that have led to the development of codes of conduct and guidance, together with requirements to conduct ethical reviews of research involving human subjects. An overarching aim of ethical review is to protect the rights, health and well-being of research participants, utilising an approach that is sensitive to diversity, cultural values and the social and cultural context in which research is conducted. Ethical principles of respect for autonomy, beneficence, non-maleficence and justice are examined and applied to the research context as a basis for decision making. Characteristics of vulnerable groups and special considerations that can apply to their participation in research are considered. Recent developments in the arena of research governance frameworks, intended to provide accountability for the moral acceptability, scientific quality and safety of research, are also briefly reviewed.

## Introduction

Research can be defined as a process of systematic enquiry involving human subjects past, present or future. In considering the moral imperative for research, few would argue with the benefits that have accrued from improvements in prophylactic, diagnostic and therapeutic procedures, the eradication of some diseases, together with improvements in quality and duration of life. The World Medical Association Declaration of Helsinki principles encapsulate key ethical principles of respect for autonomy, beneficence, non-maleficence and justice relating to medical research involving human subjects, emphasising that research is subject to ethical standards that promote respect for participants, protect their health and promote their rights:

> In medical research on human subjects, considerations relating to the well-being of the human subject should take precedence over the interests of science and society. (World Medical Association Declaration of Helsinki, 2002, principle 5)

> Every medical research project involving human subjects should be preceded by careful assessment of predictable risks and burdens in comparison with foreseeable benefits to the subject or to others. This does not preclude the participation of health volunteers in medical research. The design of all studies should be publicly available. (World Medical Association Declaration of Helsinki, 2002, principle 16)

In the conduct of research, it is vital that any foreseeable risks to the participant, whether physical, psychological or social, are removed, human dignity maintained and rights respected. Frameworks relating to human rights, for example the European Convention on Human Rights and Fundamental Freedoms enshrined in legislation within the 1998 UK Human Rights Act, also implicitly enshrine key ethical principles that inform research conduct. Articles 3, 8 and 9 are particularly relevant to minimising risks, ensuring respect for autonomy in obtaining consent to take part in research, maintaining privacy, anonymity and confidentiality for research participants.

## Historical context of research ethics

Attempts to regulate the conduct of research have a long history. Many regulations, including the earliest, have been written in response to various episodes of abuse in the name of research. Public outcry at the abuse of human rights in the Nazi concentration camps led to the Nuremberg Code (1947); however, abuse of prisoners is not confined to the Nazi regime. Many countries have documented events involving unethical conduct by mainstream medical researchers:

- The Tuskegee Syphilis Study, which began in the 1930s and continued for 42 years, used poor uneducated African American men as study subjects. The outcry to this study led to the Belmont Report and the US National Research Act (Jones, 1993).

- The vulnerability of older people to research abuse was highlighted in 1963, when it was discovered that a physician at the Jewish Chronic Disease Hospital in Brooklyn, New York, was experimentally injecting live cancer cells into elderly debilitated patients without proper informed consent (Katz, 1972). The subsequent inquiry led to the earliest European research ethics committees (RECs) being established.

- In the UK, the recent Royal Liverpool Children's Inquiry (2001) into unauthorised post-mortem removal of organs and tissues from children raised major public concerns that have resulted in new legislation, the 2004 Human Tissue Act, which regulates research on tissues and organs from live or deceased individuals.

## Ethical principles and theories

Research in human subjects is a moral endeavour, based on ethical principles of respect for autonomy, beneficence, non-maleficence and justice as fairness. Gillon (2003) has argued that recourse to these principles can "explain and justify, alone or in combination, all the substantive and universalisable claims of medical ethics and probably of ethics more generally" (p 307). Harris (2005) concedes that while the four principles can provide a useful "checklist for ethics committees without substantial ethical expertise approaching new problems" (p 303), adhering solely to the four principles could lead to sterility and uniformity of approach; analysis of arguments relevant to specific issues is vitally important in finding solutions.

## Autonomy

Autonomy is the "capacity to think, decide and act on the basis of thought and decision freely and independently" (Gillon, 1990, p 60). Respect for autonomy is justified from the consequentialist, utilitarian perspective of Mill in relation to liberty, which advocates the sovereignty or self-rule of the individual over those aspects of life that do not harm others (Himmelfarb, 1985). In contrast, the Kantian perspective requires us to "act in such a way that you treat humanity, whether in your own person or in the person of any other, never simply as a means, but always at the same time as an end" (Kant, cited by Paton, 1966, p 91). In relation to participation in research, this means it is only morally acceptable to use someone as a means to an end if they share that end and consent to it. Furthermore, unless consent is informed, the participant is used as a means, which violates autonomy.

Thus, respect for autonomy requires that individuals have the right to decide on the basis of adequate, written information and time for reflection to weigh risks and benefits and ask questions, whether or not to participate in a research study. In UK case law, consent should be given by an individual with the mental capacity to do so; information provided must be adequate and understood; consent must be freely given without coercion. Elements of informed consent include the following:

- a full explanation of the purpose of the investigation, its duration and the commitment required of participants in relation to time;
- the information to be obtained during the research and its application; use of any special procedures which may entail discomfort;
- information on potential, foreseeable risks and benefits of taking part;
- emphasis that taking part is entirely voluntary and that participants may withdraw at any time without giving reasons and without prejudice to treatment;
- in the case of therapeutic research, details of alternative treatments that exist; in non-therapeutic research an explanation of potential future benefits to others;
- information and assurances on confidentiality, anonymity, data protection and storage (1998 Data Protection Act), and access to information, for example, in the UK, interview schedules under the 2000 Freedom of Information Act;
- information relating to contact details of research personnel to clarify any matter should the need arise;
- information relating to REC approval;
- arrangements for insurance indemnity relating to the research;
- details of the information that will be supplied to participants during the study; this can include interim and concluding findings.

Details of the research sponsor and funding body should also be provided. Informed consent is an ongoing requirement, thus researchers must ascertain that participants "continue to consent and understand the elements of informed consent outlined above; this includes any changes in information" (Royal College of Nursing, 2005, p 3).

In gaining informed consent, researchers must respect diversity and consider culture, ethnicity, gender, disability, religious beliefs, language and understanding (Nuffield Council on Bioethics, 2002; DH, 2005).

Language used in the preparation of information sheets for potential participants should avoid medical jargon and be clearly comprehensible to the lay person; feedback from the lay representative on the REC can be invaluable here. Information may need presenting in different formats to meet the needs of potential participants with regard to language, disability and impairment; use of professional interpreters may be necessary. Stead et al (2005) used focus groups to identify the interpretation and understanding of prospective participants in randomised controlled clinical trials in relation to use of concepts such as 'randomisation' and 'double-blinding'. Findings were that respondents had problems comprehending these concepts and found them threatening in relation to care. Stead et al (2005) emphasised that the quality of communication between the person taking consent and the potential participant was intrinsic to valid consent, that written information should explain why randomisation is necessary, why it is important to avoid bias and why doctors should not be involved in the randomisation process.

It is also important that time is allowed for individuals to ask questions to clarify any matter and that consent is accurately documented in relation to understanding of the issues and agreement to taking part. Usually, written consent is required, but verbal consent can be acceptable in certain circumstances, for example with the support of an independent witness, if the participant cannot sign a consent form due to physical disability (see implied consent below). Some types of research may require non-disclosure of information to avoid bias, for example, covert observation of human behaviour or interactions in an outpatients clinic waiting room. This type of research is frequently justified on the basis that it exposes the participant to minimum risk, does not breach privacy and there are benefits that accrue to society. For further information on covert, observational research, see the professional guidelines of The British Psychological Society (2003) (www.bps.org.uk/index.cfm) and The British Sociological Association (2002) (www.britsoc.co.uk).

In certain circumstances it may not be possible to obtain participants' consent before research commences, for example in Accident and Emergency situations. The 2005 Mental Capacity Act states that research can be undertaken in these circumstances if "it is not reasonably practical" to obtain informed consent due to lack of capacity. However, the researchers should subsequently obtain informed consent from the participant as soon as it is possible to do so. Implied consent refers to situations where a potential participant cannot either write or verbally communicate their consent, usually due to injuries or disability. Relevant criteria that apply are that the person can be reasonably expected to understand information, is provided with a means of withholding consent and does not do so and benefits outweigh risks. Here, consent can be obtained in the presence of a witness who is then required to sign the consent form.

Under the 2005 Mental Capacity Act (for implementation in 2007), it will be possible for another person to give informed consent for an incapacitated adult to take part in a research study; advance directives will be considered in decision making. For detailed information relating to issues of consent in vulnerable groups (children, pregnant women, people with learning disabilities, unresponsive patients) the reader is directed to the 1989 Children Act, the 1991 Age of Legal Capacity (Scotland) Act, the 2000 Adults with Incapacity Act (Scotland), the 2004 Medicines for Human Use (Clinical Trials) Regulations, the 2005 Mental Capacity Act, Council for International Organisations of Medical Sciences (CIOMS) (1993), Royal College of Paediatrics and Child Health (2000) and General Medical Council (GMC) (2002).

## Beneficence, non-maleficence

The principle of beneficence requires that researchers act to promote the well-being of participants; the principle of non-maleficence that they do no harm. In the UK, civil law also requires researchers to exercise a duty of care to participants and liability can arise for damage, injury or death caused by acts or omissions, the results of which should have been reasonably foreseeable. Taking part in research can benefit participants in diverse ways, for example by "accessing treatments that may give better outcomes than standard treatments available; closer monitoring; increased access to a multidisciplinary team; altruistic satisfactions of benefiting future patients" and volunteers may also benefit financially (Royal College of Nursing, 2004, p 9). Potential risks to participants can arise from invasive biological or psychological techniques, drug toxicity and allergic reactions in randomised trials, interviewing on sensitive subjects, loss of privacy, time or financial resources.

The principles of beneficence and non-maleficence require what is essentially a consequentialist weighing of risks versus benefits to participants to be completed, that is, a risk assessment. Participants (see above), researchers and independent RECs need to evaluate and weigh potential benefits and risks. Normally, risks to participants should not exceed minimal risk, that is, that ordinarily encountered in daily life; this assumes such risks are known, quantifiable and that this threshold is clearly defined. Kopelman (2004) has drawn attention to the different interpretations of minimal risk in many countries. In considering the need to exercise beneficence and non-maleficence, the following should be considered:

- Researchers need to work within their expertise and competence; training in any techniques should be provided before the start of a research study to satisfy governance requirements.
- If emerging findings could pose a risk to participant well-being, the REC and participants should be informed.
- Factors that might exacerbate risk should be fully evaluated before commencing a study, for example pre-existing medical conditions.
- Researchers need to be aware of situations that can arise, often unexpectedly, and require an intervention on ethical grounds to safeguard participant welfare.
- Participation in research can raise anxieties and concerns; provision of debriefing sessions that allow participants to discuss and resolve these are helpful. In some circumstances referral for specialist help may be necessary if the researcher cannot resolve the problem.
- Sensitivity to cultural values and an awareness of the social and cultural context in which research is conducted is vital (Nuffield Council on Bioethics, 2002).
- Researchers should be aware of threats to their own safety and well-being that can arise in the conduct of social research (The British Sociological Association professional guidelines, 2002, www.britsoc.co.uk).

Increasingly, in randomised controlled clinical trials, data monitoring committees (DMCs) are playing a role in evaluating interim evidence related to benefits and toxicity. Recommendations made can require modification of a study protocol or early termination of a study (Artinian et al, 2004). Currently, the remit of DMCs is developmental and while general agreement exists that a DMC should be independent and multidisciplinary, consumer and ethicist membership is controversial (Grant et al, 2005). Also controversial is a broader DMC role in relation to ethical issues that are currently within the remit of RECs.

## Justice

The principle of justice as fairness is widely acknowledged in research ethics, both from an Aristotelian perspective that equals ought to be considered equally (Thomson, 1966) and that of the theory of justice outlined by Rawls (1976). In the latter, it is proposed that "each individual has an equal right to the most extensive basic liberty compatible with a single liberty for others and that social and economic inequalities are to be arranged so that they are reasonably expected to be to everyone's advantage" (p 60). Fair, equitable treatment of research participants can encompass the following:

- non-discrimination in selection of participants together with equitable sharing of risks and benefits;
- respecting participants' rights not to take part and to withdraw from a research study without prejudice;
- ensuring that any financial agreements are honoured and adherence to ethically approved research protocols is maintained;
- respecting and maintaining confidentiality of information, rights to privacy and anonymity, requirements for secure data storage and protection.

Significant controversy involving considerations of justice as fairness and beneficence have arisen in relation to the standards of care that pertain to participants in randomised, controlled clinical trials conducted in developing countries. Principle 29 of the World Medical Association Declaration of Helsinki (2002, 2004) recommends that "... benefits, risks, burdens and effectiveness of a new method should be tested against those of the best current prophylactic, diagnostic, and therapeutic methods. This does not exclude the use of placebo, or no treatment, in studies where no proven prophylactic, diagnostic or therapeutic method exists".

Furthermore, principle 30, recommends that at the conclusion of a trial, every patient entered should be assured of "... access to the best proven prophylactic, diagnostic and therapeutic methods...". In developing countries, standards of care do not approach those in more affluent locations and very few options for therapy may exist; how then to ensure justice in treating people equally?

Recommendations of the Nuffield Council on Bioethics (2002) are that "wherever possible, participants in a control group should be offered a universal standard of care and where this is not possible the minimum standard that should be offered to the control group is the best intervention for that disease as part of the national public health system" (p xv). Emphasis is also placed on the need for decisions to be made before trials begin about interventions to be offered to control groups on conclusion and that information relating to this should be provided in obtaining informed consent from participants. Researchers are recommended to secure post-trial access for effective interventions for participants before commencing a study and to justify the lack of provision to an REC. Conflicting statements of the World Medical Association, the Nuffield Council on Bioethics and other bodies highlight the difficulties in reaching a consensus, concerns about exploitation and the acceptability of views that justice does not always require all people to be treated the same (Lie et al, 2003; McMillan and Conlon, 2004).

## Vulnerable research participants

Some of the most egregious research studies have consistently targeted specific groups of people considered in some way to be inferior. In most cases these people are more vulnerable than other members of our communities. Prisoners and other people who live in circumstances best described in the terms by the Australian National Health and Medical Research Council as *dependent or unequal relationships* are particularly vulnerable to exploitation and abuse (National Health and Medical Research Council, 1999). The requirement of first-person voluntary informed consent is particularly important with regard to people living in dependent or unequal relationships, because the potential of abuse is greater. Characteristics of the vulnerable and devalued populations as potential research subjects can be identified:

- their circumstances put them at risk for loss of decision-making capacity. This can be either through aetiology of disease, developmental delay, or socially induced;
- they are likely to be economically/socially disadvantaged;
- they are little understood, often demeaned, and unjustifiably feared. With many of the vulnerable populations used there is, or has been, a stigma attached to membership of that group.

Inability to adequately engage in the process of voluntary and informed consent – for whatever reasons – raises the research participant's degree of risk and vulnerability:

> Competent but vulnerable adults may find it difficult to withhold consent if they are put under implicit or explicit pressures from institutions or health care professionals. But the treatments being researched might be of significant benefit to such people, and to exclude vulnerable groups could be a form of discrimination. Frail elderly people, people living in institutions and adults with learning difficulties or mental illness who remain competent should all be considered vulnerable. Pregnant women may also be subjected to hidden pressures to become involved in research, and their inclusion in a project may need special consideration. (GMC, 2002, principle 43)

A protectionist stance that shields vulnerable groups from research participation may deny them the benefits garnered from scientific research that are available to other populations. Paradoxically, such exclusion may reinforce their vulnerability. When diseases that affect women, minorities and other undervalued populations are not addressed by research, knowledge that could rectify prevailing ineffectual or harmful routine medical care is never produced (Dresser, 1992; Charo, 1993).

## Impact and influence of research regulation

### Research design

> The experiment should be so designed and based on the results of animal experimentation and a knowledge of the natural history of the disease or other problem under study that the anticipated results will justify the performance of the experiment. (Nuremberg Code, 1947, no 3)

> Scientifically unsound research on human subjects is ipso facto unethical in that it may expose subjects to risk or inconvenience to no purpose. (CIOMS, 1993, no 14, commentary)

These are typical expressions of the ethical requirement that research must be sufficiently well designed to achieve its purposes; otherwise, it is not justified. The primary principle of this norm is to uphold the principle of beneficence. If research is not well designed, there will be no benefits; investigators who conduct badly designed research are not responsive to the obligation to do good or to develop generalisable knowledge that is sufficiently important to justify the risks of physical or psychological harms imposed on human subjects.

## Competence of the investigator

This norm requires that the investigators be competent in at least two respects. They should have adequate scientific training and skill to accomplish the purposes of the research. The purpose of this component of the norm is precisely the same as that requiring good research design; it is responsive primarily to the obligations to produce benefits to society through the development of important knowledge. It is also responsive to the obligation to show respect for research participants by not wasting their time or frustrating their wishes to participate in meaningful activities. In addition investigators are expected to be sufficiently competent to care for the subject. The Declaration of Helsinki, as an instrument of the World Medical Association, is addressed only to medical research. Therefore, it places responsibility with "… a medically qualified person". The Nuremberg Code (1947), on the other hand, is addressed more generally to research; consequently, it does not call for medical qualification.

Regulation not only protects participants in research, but it also protects researchers. It sets out clearly what is acceptable and what is not, and therefore provides a framework within which researchers work. The central tenet of the Hippocratic oath is that the primary obligation of physicians is to benefit their patients. This fundamental ethic recognises the patient's potential for vulnerability and thus requires that physicians act solely on behalf of their patients' best interests.

## Scrutiny and regulation of research

The international codes and regulations that were developed after the Nuremberg Code (1947) have attempted to reconcile society's twin responsibilities to adequately protect vulnerable research participants and to ensure that vulnerable populations receive the benefits of research. The various drafts of the World Medical Association Declaration of Helsinki, first issued in 1964, have endeavoured to ease the consent requirements for people who lack capacity to consent to research. The Declaration classifies research as *therapeutic* and *non-therapeutic* (World Medical Association Declaration of Helsinki, 1964). The *International ethical guidelines for biomedical research involving human subjects*, which also considers, among other concerns, research involving people who are incapable of giving adequately informed consent, was issued by CIOMS in collaboration with the World Health Organisation (WHO) (CIOMS, 1993).

Within the UK the regulation applying to biomedical research derives from a number of sources:

- *Statute:* Acts of Parliament (primary legislation, which could include directly applicable European Union law) may prohibit certain activities or may require certain conditions to be met before activities can take place. Different statutes cover different parts of the UK, and different parts of the UK may interpret EU legislation differently. The likelihood of this occurring has increased with devolution. For example, most of the 2004 Human Tissue Act does not apply in Scotland. Such variation can present problems for researchers who move within the UK and also for cross-border collaborations.
- *Common law:* principles contained within case law, such as the nature and meaning of informed consent or the duty of care, can impose requirements on the conduct of research.
- *Secondary legislation:* these are rules made under statutory authority and approved by Parliament, including provisions implementing obligations arising from EU directives.
- *Administrative rules, including self-regulation:* rules or guidance may come from government departments, professional bodies and employers or funders. Such rules do not have the formal effect of law but may impose real obligations on researchers.

The UK has no single, national ethics committee that undertakes research appraisal. Instead, there is a centrally administered system of regional ethics committees that assess any research on humans that uses NHS patients or resources or that accesses participants via the NHS. The scrutiny of non-NHS research remains the responsibility of the funding body or host institution.

## Research in the NHS

Ethical scrutiny of research involving human subjects in the NHS is undertaken by a system of RECs. The Central Office for Research Ethics Committees (COREC) was established by the Department of Health in 1997 to provide operational support and advice to NHS RECs. In 2001, COREC issued the *Governance arrangements for NHS research ethics committees* (GafREC). These define the remit and accountability of RECs, and give guidance on membership and the process of ethical review.

The EU Clinical Trials Directive (2004) regulates clinical trials. This requires a single ethical opinion to be given on a clinical trial in any member state. In 2004, the UK Ethics Committee Authority (UKECA), composed of UK health ministers, was created as the body responsible for establishing, recognising and monitoring RECs to review clinical trials of medicines under the Directive. UKECA has recognised a number of (mostly NHS) RECs to review clinical trials proposals; COREC acts for UKECA in providing advice/assistance to these committees. In 2004, COREC introduced standard operating procedures (SOPs) for NHS RECs. The SOPs implement the requirements of the Directive. Only one REC application is now required for any clinical trial. COREC decided that the SOPs should also apply to all other NHS research reviewed by NHS RECs.

## Non-NHS research

Clinical trials in private facilities are required by law to receive approval from a recognised REC. The NHS RECs may review other private sector research on people, although there is no statutory obligation to do this. Many proposals will still pass through institutional ethics committees that may vary widely in their remit, membership and process. Currently there is no equivalent supervisory body as COREC for non-NHS RECs. Many universities now have their own ethics committees that scrutinise research proposals: a recent study found that 80% of UK universities have their own REC (Tinker and Coomber, 2004). Major funders of research, such as the Medical Research Council (MRC) and Cancer Research UK, require that proposals for research involving people, data or tissue, receive a favourable opinion from an REC before funding is provided.

## Social research

Social research that involves NHS resources, facilities, staff or data must be subject to review by the NHS REC system. Non-NHS projects may have to be approved by university or institutional ethics committees, although there is no statutory requirement for this. Social and psychological researchers have emphasised the need for ethical review of their research in order to retain public confidence, and participation, in projects. Recent years have also seen an increase in the use of social research data in policy, which has led to an increased awareness of the need for good ethical and professional research practice. Until recently there were few attempts to formulate a single ethical code for social research. However, this has changed with the recent developments outlined below:

- publication of the Department of Health's Social Care Implementation Plan and the Department for Work and Pensions' mission statement outlining its approach to ethical issues in research;
- pending publication of the government Social Research Unit's framework for ethical assurance of government-commissioned social research, intended to ensure consistency of standards in social research across government departments. The Scottish Executive is currently conducting a similar review;
- publication of the Economic and Social Research Council's *Developing a framework for social science research ethics* (ESRC, 2005).

## Ethics review of social care research

The *Research governance framework* (DH, 2005) requires that an independent review is undertaken of all health and social care research (see Chapter Four, this volume). A current challenge is that there is no system for review of social care research comparable to that undertaken by NHS RECs. While social care research involving NHS staff and users is covered by the NHS RECs, it is acknowledged that a considerable volume of social care research would not be appropriate for review by NHS RECs, notably that involving social care agencies and populations (DH, 2004). In acknowledgement that a system for ethics review in social care will need to be developed, an option appraisal and consultation exercise has been undertaken. Potential models proposed for a more comprehensive review of social care research include a national system of RECs similar to the NHS REC modus operandi, a committee system operating within the established COREC structures, a national system for social care ethics review and a pluralist system based on local diversity. Currently, the outcome of the consultation exercise on these models or other feasible alternatives is awaited.

## Complexity of ethical review

In conjunction with the inception of research governance, an increasing number of health care organisations have written guidelines on the conduct of research. This has not always been to the advantage of the research process resulting in, at times, a more restricting research environment, rather than one of greater awareness and understanding. The answers to ensuring that research involving human participants is conducted ethically may, however, lie elsewhere: in ensuring that researchers understand their ethical obligations when undertaking research and in ensuring that ethics review committees are adequately supported to provide the necessary oversight.

Within the UK the system for ethical review of research involving humans is complex and varies considerably between medical, social and psychological research. In relation to the new arrangements for research governance, a clear need exists to reduce the complexity and to improve the coordination of the system. In addition, concerns have been raised about inconsistent ethical standards, inappropriate ethical review, lack of transparency, coordination and efficiency of the various ethical review systems and negative impacts on the costs and dissemination of research. New governance frameworks in development should ensure that duplication of ethical scrutiny is avoided and rationalise arrangements for approvals (Holmes, 2004; Medical Research Council, 2004).

## Conclusions and contemporary challenges for research

Ethical research promotes respect for the health, well-being and rights of voluntary participants and, in its conduct, foreseeable risks should be removed and dignity maintained. Ethical principles of respect for autonomy, beneficence, non-maleficence and justice provide a basis for decision making and ethical reviews of research. Contemporary challenges in research ethics encompass the continuing need to protect vulnerable groups, to consider the implications of externally funded research in developing countries and to provide rigorous ethical regulation that avoids bureaucracy and over-complexity.

## References

Adults Incapacity Act (Scotland) 2000, London: The Stationery Office (www.scotland-legislation.hmso.gov.uk/legislation/scotland).

Age of Legal Capacity Act (Scotland) 1991, London: HMSO (www.scotland-legislation.hmso.gov.uk/legislation/scotland).

Artinian, N.T., Froelicher, E.S. and Vander Wal, J.S. (2004) 'Data and safety monitoring during randomised controlled trials of nursing interventions', *Nursing Research*, vol 53, no 6, pp 414-18.

Charo, A. (1993) 'Protecting us to death: women, pregnancy, and clinical research trials', *Health Law Symposium*, vol 38, pp 135-67.

Children Act 1989, London: HMSO (www.opsi.gov.uk/acts/acts1989/Ukpga_19890041_en_1.htm).

CIOMS (Council for International Organisations of Medical Sciences) in collaboration with WHO (World Health Organisation) (1993) 'International ethical guidelines for biomedical research involving human subjects', in H. Vanderpool (ed) *The ethics of research involving human subjects: Facing the 21st century*, Frederick, MA: University Publishing Group, pp 501-10.

Data Protection Act 1998, London: The Stationery Office (www.opsi.gov.uk/acts/acts1998/19980029.htm).

DH (Department of Health) (2004) *Ethics review of social care research: Options appraisal and guidelines* (www.dh.gov.uk/consultations).

DH (2005) *Research governance framework for health and social care* (2nd edn), London: DH.

Dresser, R. (1992) 'Wanted: single, white male for medical research', *Hastings Center Report*, vol 22, no 1, pp 24-9.

ESRC (Economic and Social Research Council) (2005) *Developing a framework for social science research ethics* (www.york.ac.uk/res/ref).

EU (European Union) Clinical Trials Directive (2004) (www.mrc.ac.uk/index/current-research/current-clinical_research/funding-clinical_research_governance/current-eu_clinical_trials_directive.htm).

Freedom of Information Act 2000, London: The Stationery Office (www.opsi.gov.uk/acts/acts2000/20000036.htm).

Gillon, R. (1990) *Philosophical medical ethics*, Chichester: John Wiley.

Gillon, R. (2003) 'Ethics needs principles – four can encompass the rest – and respect for autonomy should be first among equals', *Journal of Medical Ethics*, vol 29, pp 307-12.

GMC (General Medical Council) (2002) *Research: The role and responsibilities of doctors*, London: GMC Publications.

Grant, A.M., Altman, D.G. and Babiker, A.B. (2005) 'Issues in data monitoring and interim analysis of trials', *Health Technology Assessment*, vol 9, no 7, pp 1-238.

Harris, J. (2005) 'Scientific research is a moral duty', *Journal of Medical Ethics*, vol 31, pp 242-8.

Himmelfarb, G. (1985) *On liberty*, London: Penguin.

Holmes, S. (2004) 'Is governance now inhibiting research?', *British Journal of Healthcare Management*, vol 10, pp 305-9.

Human Rights Act 1998, London, The Stationery Office (www.opsi.gov.uk/acts/acts1998/19980042.htm).

Human Tissue Act 2004, London, The Stationery Office (www.opsi.gov.uk/acts/acts2004/20040030.htm).

Jones, J.H. (1993) *Bad blood: The Tuskegee Syphilis Experiment*, New York, NY: Free Press.

Katz, J. (1972) *Experiments with human bodies*, New York, NY: Russell Sage.

Kopelman, L.M. (2004) 'Minimal risk as an international ethical standard in research', *Journal of Medical Philosophy*, vol 29, no 3, pp 351-78.

Lie, R.K., Emanuel, E., Grady, C. and Wendler, D. (2003) 'The standard of care debate: the Declaration of Helsinki versus the international consensus opinion', *Journal of Medical Ethics*, vol 30, pp 190-3.

McMillan, J.R. and Conlon, C. (2004) 'The ethics of research related to healthcare in developing countries', *Journal of Medical Ethics*, vol 30, pp 204-6.

Medical Research Council (2004) *Position statement on research regulation and ethics*, London: Medical Research Council Publications.

Mental Capacity Act 2005, London, The Stationery Office (www.opsi.gov.uk/acts/acts2004/20040030.htm).

Mental Capacity Bill Draft Code of Practice (2005), London: The Stationery Office (www.dca.gov.uk/menincap/mcbdraftcode.pdf).

National Health and Medical Research Council (1999) *National statement on ethical conduct in research involving humans*, Canberra, Australia: AusInfo.

Nuffield Council on Bioethics (2002) *The ethics of research related to healthcare in developing countries*, London: Nuffield Council on Bioethics Publications.

Nuremberg Code (1947) (http://ohsr.od.nih.gov/guidelines/nuremberg.html), reprinted from *Trials of war criminals before the Nuremberg Military Tribunals under Control Council Law No 10, Vol 2, pp 181-182*, Washington, DC: US Government Printing Office, 1949.

Paton, H.J. (1966) *The moral law*, London: Hutchinson University Library.

Rawls, J. (1976) *A theory of justice*, Oxford: Oxford University Press.

Royal College of Nursing (2004) *Research ethics*, London: Royal College of Nursing.

Royal College of Nursing (2005) *Informed consent in health and social care research*, London: Royal College of Nursing.

Royal College of Paediatrics and Child Health (2000) 'Guidelines for the ethical conduct of medical research in children', *Archives of Disease in Childhood*, vol 82, no 2, pp 177-82.

Royal Liverpool Children's Inquiry, The (2001) London: The Stationery Office (www.rlcinquiry.org.uk/download/index.htm).

Stead, M., Eadie, D., Gordon, D. and Angus, K. (2005) '"Hello, hello – it's English I speak!": a qualitative exploration of patients' understanding of the science of clinical trials', *Journal of Medical Ethics*, vol 31, pp 664-9.

Thomson, J.A.K. (1966) *The ethics of Aristotle*, London: Penguin.

Tinker, A. and Coomber, V. (2004) 'University research ethics committees: their role, remit and conduct', *Bulletin of Medical Ethics*, vol 11, pp 7-8.

World Medical Association Declaration of Helsinki (1964, 2002, 2004) *Ethical principles for medical research involving human subjects* (www.wma.net/e/policy/b3.htm).

# FOUR

# Ethics: research governance for health and social care

*Elaine Pierce*

## Summary

Research and Development (R&D) in health and social care is dependent on funding from government or charitable sources, public confidence and concrete support. Therefore it is essential that R&D be conducted according to regulations that are both stringent and transparent. In the UK, R&D, carried out by organisations and individuals, is subject to the *Research governance framework for health and social care* (DH, 2005). This framework, which is overseen by the relevant government department, aims to enhance the promotion and quality of R&D and to ensure a sustainable research culture. Research governance compliance criteria include the need for independent scientific review of the research proposal; ethical approval; and sponsorship and supervision by responsible health and social care professionals. The ethical implications of the patient's autonomy and consent within the framework, alongside those of monitoring, accountability, leadership and management, will be examined in this chapter. Shortcomings in the conduct of R&D and subsequent evidence-based practice will also be considered.

## Introduction

The World Health Organisation (WHO) urges countries to create a climate in which research for health will flourish. It proposes universal ethical standards, a wider view of health with more civil society involvement and more financial investment from governments (WHO, 2004). Research governance is not unique to the UK. Governance in some form or another is undertaken in a number of countries throughout the world. According to Alexander et al (2003), health research governance should include the plan for setting and monitoring organisational goals and developing strategies by a board of trustees or directors, to which the chief administrator reports. In the UK, the *Research governance framework for health and social care* is implemented through a strategic plan developed by the board within the R&D department at the Department of Health (DH) and the reporting administrator to this board is the responsible person in a hospital's R&D department.

In research, as in other aspects of care, all individuals have rights in order to protect them and maintain their confidentiality (DH, 1995; 1998 Data Protection Act; 1998 Human Rights Act). Abuse of these rights can lead to litigation. Research governance creates a climate in which research can be carried out without contravening an individual's rights. This is done through assigning roles and responsibilities to all involved, encompassing researchers, funders, research sponsors, care organisations and formal carers. It is also intended to prevent misconduct and fraud. Thus the framework "provides guidance on good practice in the collaboration between researchers, health and social care agencies and research funders" and defines research as "the attempt to derive generalisable new knowledge by addressing clearly defined questions with systematic and rigorous methods" (DH, 2005, p 3).

This very clear and poignant definition would be futile and meaningless unless research findings are shared with fellow health and social care professionals, policy and decision makers, the wider scientific community and service users in general. The *World report on knowledge for better health* emphasises the importance of sharing appropriate and valid research information. It is referred to as the 'know–do gap', where pathways are created for the effective translation, transfer and use of the evidence in practice (WHO, 2004). All involved should, therefore, aim not only to conduct good research, but also to maximise opportunities for getting the evidence to the shop floor, where it would be most relevant.

The research governance framework can be traced to the DH strategy *Research and development for a first class service* (2000). The first edition of the *Research governance framework* was published in 2001 (DH, 2001); the second edition (2005) puts more emphasis on attempts to make clearer criticisms of the initial framework, especially in relation to responsibilities and accountability. It is important for all individuals, consumers, carers, researchers, students and health and social care professionals and organisations, whether directly or indirectly under the responsibility of the Secretary of State for Health, to adhere to the framework. In this chapter 'protocol' and 'proposals' are used synonymously and 'health care professional' refers to both qualified and unqualified staff working in the UK's National Health Service (NHS), social services or their contracted agencies or in independent or charitable health organisations, which receive funding from the DH to support their research programme. 'Researcher' refers to an investigator, whether they be the chief/lead, principal or other investigator. 'Organisation' refers to the NHS, their research partners, social services or their contracted agencies and organisations or institutions receiving DH funding as above.

## Legislation, regulations and standards

Legislation, regulations, standards and guidance are all about improving the quality of research and safeguarding and promoting the rights, dignity and well-being of individuals, mainly the research participants. In the light of adverse events such as The Bristol Infirmary Inquiry (2001) and The Royal Liverpool Children's Inquiry (2001) there has been new legislation. The 2004 Human Tissue Act, which comes into effect in 2006, deals with consent for research on tissues and organs from live or post-mortem individuals, their storage and disposal in a respectful manner. The 2005 Mental Capacity Act, which comes into force in 2007, conserves the rights of the mentally incapacitated individual. This Act also stipulates that a body, usually a Research Ethics Committee (REC), must review an incapacitated individual's previous wishes, interests and feelings, and that researchers follow the statutory code of practice in relation to consent. The research governance framework (DH, 2005) outlines an example of good practice, which upholds a participant's rights in research. Other changes include regulation on clinical trials of medicines, for example, the 2004 Medicines for Human Use (Clinical Trials) Regulations provides for informed consent and the recruitment of minors and incapacitated adults. Section 60 of the 2001 Health and Social Care Act legislates the only occasions when information that will identify an individual can be used without consent.

The Home Office enforces strict controls where essential research can only be undertaken using animals and in this case numerous licences are required (the 1996 Animals (Scientific Procedures) Act 1986 (Appropriate Methods of Humane Killing) Order). There is no equivalent for licensing, in spite of the framework, of individuals undertaking research on human participants, their body parts or tissues. Therefore, the ethical supervision of human research should be more stringent, with formal training to improve understanding of research methods and ethics and licensing of researchers (Jamrozik, 2000, 2004).

The majority of researchers in health and social services are professionals, who can be held accountable for their actions. In engaging in research they are not only governed by their own professional codes of conduct and standards but also by the research governance framework. Many professional associations, societies and unions have forums, sub-groups or committees that deal with specific areas such as research (BPS, 2004; Royal College of Nursing, 2004; BMA, 2005; NHS R&D Forum, 2006). In most cases the role of these research forums or sub-groups is to act as a source of help, information and support educationally and often financially, in the form of awards, grants or bursaries, too. Hence, they produce standards/guidance relating to ethical conduct and source materials, and organise courses and conferences. These are generally available for all their members and at times are also open to non-members. Since the membership consists of ordinary grass-roots professionals who are either actively involved with, engaging in, or have a general interest in research, they are the most suitable for debating and problem solving. It is also these groups that are utilised when, for example, the DH and others approach the association or organisation for consultation. Associations and unions also often have a dedicated web page for research.

"RG [research governance] is one of the core standards for health care organisations" (DH, 2005, p ii). Hence, they must have systems in place that meet and ensure the consistent application of the framework. This also relates to their Duty of Quality as stated in section 45 of the 2003 Health and Social Care (Community Health and Standards) Act. All research has to adhere to the framework; however, because of differences in the nature and quantity of research, funding, stakeholders, academic disciplines and delivery methods in social care compared to the NHS, changes in the introduction and implementation of a social care research governance framework had to be made (DH, 2004a).

According to the *Implementation plan for social care* (DH, 2004a), unlike health care research, the majority of participants recruited to social care research are from the most socioeconomically deprived and marginalised areas of society. This poses different risks and problems. For example, the research can be regarded as intrusive, some may find it distressing and it can have an adverse effect on well-being. Other differences relate to the type and quantity of research, the structure of the local service and the mix of stakeholders and academic disciplines. It is also possible that research governance and culture in social care

are not as evenly advanced as in the NHS, because of the numerous agencies (statutory and independent) involved. The research governance framework is applicable to social services (adult and child) or their contracted agencies, but not automatically to data obtained from another source or department within the council. For example, the framework does not cover housing and education (DH, 2004a). This could lead to problems where there is overlap or where individuals or agencies have to make decisions as to whether the framework is relevant. There has been consultation on a national ethics system for social care, similar to that of the NHS RECs, with the Association of Directors of Social Services (Dolan et al, 2004) favouring a system parallel to that of the NHS, provided it is acceptable to the majority of social care research stakeholders.

## Research governance framework

In theory, the sentiments that provoked the formation of the research governance framework are very laudable, especially in relation to the roles of the sponsor, protection of participants and accountability of researchers. In practice, however, interpreting, implementing and maintaining certain aspects can be difficult. The bureaucracy of the framework could prevent the uptake of research (Holmes, 2004; SDO News, 2005). For example, to avoid the lengthy processes intrinsic to the research governance framework, health professionals may choose to engage in audit instead of research (Duffin, 2005; Samanta and Samanta, 2005). The care home sector, whose status can be both private or public, poses particular issues: for example, are the clients tenants or receivers of care, since each presents different rights for the individuals and responsibilities for the care home (Reed et al, 2004)? There could also be variation in terms of data protection, criminal record checks on researchers and provision of honorary contracts to researchers at organisations that are not their employers. Some organisations deal with such matters very rapidly, while others are not so efficient and may take weeks or months to finalise arrangements (Duffin, 2005).

Awareness of the framework may also vary within and between organisations. Smith et al (2005) found no statistical difference in awareness between staff that had been trained in research governance and researchers, but significant differences between these two groups and staff who were non-researchers or untrained. Their results also show that generally staff felt the approval process to be too complicated. While some recognised the importance of research, the majority said they did not have time to engage in it. Promotion of the research governance framework is so important that some feel it should be part of the induction programme for staff, especially students, and that monies should be set aside specifically for training so that researchers are adequately aware and prepared (Samanta and Samanta, 2005).

The role of the REC is to give an independent view of how a research project meets ethical standards. The UK Ethics Committee's Authority should accredit ethics committees assessing clinical trials involving medicines. No research should commence or its protocol be changed without a favourable opinion from an REC and written permission from the organisations' chief executive or their equivalent (DH, 2004b). Wainwright and Saunders (2004) argue that, since roles and responsibilities are clearly defined in the research governance framework, it should not be the remit of the REC to assess whether a researcher is competent to undertake research and whether the necessary resources are in place. They state that members of RECs do not have this local knowledge and these questions are empirical rather than ethical. The responsibility should, therefore, lie with the sponsor, the organisation and the principal investigator.

The sponsor and the funder have entirely different roles. The funder finances the research. However, there is no reason why the sponsor or the funder cannot be both. The sponsor of the research can be an individual, organisation or institution, or a group of individuals, organisations or institutions. The sponsor has an all-encompassing role from the beginning to the end of the research. They must ensure, in accordance with the research governance framework (DH, 2005):

- before the research starts, that researchers are competent, the necessary resources are available and agreements and structures are in place for monitoring, auditing, reporting, approving, funding and registering a trial, which must also meet legal requirements;
- during the research, protocol and relevant policies are adhered to, changes, adverse incidents or events are reported, participants and others are not put at risk, research is appropriately and adequately supervised and research participants are compensated if harmed;
- on completion of the research, it is properly concluded and findings disseminated as widely as possible, not only to the participants and others involved, but also to the wider community of health professionals and the general public, locally, nationally and internationally.

# Research and development

R&D departments provide a wide-ranging service (Pierce, 2003), for and on behalf of their organisation, researchers, participants, formal and informal carers, service users and support groups. This includes managing budgets funded from the DH and other awards, monitoring, supervising, auditing, advising, providing training, keeping themselves, their organisation and researchers updated on the latest developments in research, as well as producing reports such as the annual report to the DH and having signed agreements with partners in research, for example, universities and other organisations or institutions. The quality and quantity of service provision differs in R&D departments and is dependent on a number of factors, such as size of the organisation, number of staff employed, level of funding, number of researchers and research projects.

R&D departments, advisory bodies in R&D programmes, RECs, reviewers and researchers all have a responsibility in insuring that the vast array of diversity within the human population (age, disability, sexual orientation, 'race', colour, religion, etc) is respected and reflected in the research undertaken (DH, 2005).

Researchers should at all times collaborate with and keep their R&D departments fully informed. This practice should apply from the initial idea stage through the entire research process until such time that the research is deemed to be complete. What defines completion is not clear in the research governance framework and may vary between organisations. Research should only be regarded as complete once the findings have been disseminated.

The author holds the view that dissemination should be via a peer review journal, to provide the basis for evidence-based practice, through oral presentation and/or a lay information leaflet to the participants (patients, carers, relatives, service users, staff), taking into account everyone's needs, for example, where appropriate, in a language other than English, Braille or large print. In this way the information is cascaded to everyone. After all, it was the public and/or their body parts that were used in the research and the public purse that provided the funding. Researchers should be aware from the outset that all findings should be shared with others, bearing in mind the 'know–do gap' (WHO, 2004). Negative findings are still outcomes and should not be forgotten or shelved. There is also a need for committee or board members at conferences and/or scientific and professional journals to be more willing to accept for presentation and publication negative research results. Dissemination can only be regarded as ethical when all the evidence is provided.

It is also unethical as well as foolish for researchers not to consult with R&D departments, as the failure to follow research governance framework procedures could have great repercussions for a research study. For example, it could prove very costly in terms of recruitment and retention of subjects, data collection, financial implications in terms of researchers' or research assistants' time and cost incurred (Jones and Bamford, 2004). Irrespective of whether incorrect research governance framework procedures were carried out knowingly or unknowingly, if R&D departments were not informed, when found out, researchers could be left confused, stressed, demoralised, angry and less likely to do research in the future.

The research governance framework (DH, 2005) states that users, informal carers and groups representing them should whenever possible be part of the research process. Technically, they could therefore participate in all or any of the stages, from putting forward an idea and designing its protocol, through collecting and analysing data, to dissemination of the findings. R&D departments should welcome this input from non-health professionals or users since they often view research in a different light and propose ideas that may not occur to professionals. It is also useful to have these non-professionals or users on committees when proposals are being discussed.

INVOLVE, funded by the DH, is a body made up of the general public, voluntary and charitable organisations, health and social services managers and researchers, set up to 'promote public involvement in research'. They produce leaflets, a newsletter and provide training so that there is an 'active partnership' between all involved in research rather than the public being used only as participants of research.

R&D departments have a responsibility for maintaining standards and should be held accountable if they do not do so. They should provide direction and training (Samanta and Samanta, 2005) to prevent ill-informed researchers engaging in projects that are unethical or of little worth. Regular monitoring and random auditing of all researchers and research is of the utmost importance. Additionally, there should be encouragement of and support for self-reporting and whistle-blowing of adverse events and incidents. All parties are accountable and it beholds everyone to adhere strictly to the research governance framework.

There should be a random audit of 10% of research projects each year, to check, among others, the following: a valid favourable ethical opinion; funding; consent forms have been properly completed and signed; and audit may also include verification of procedures through interview or observation of a small number of participants (DH, 2002). There should also be random monitoring to assess protocols approved by the trust's approval body and those submitted to the ethics committee are not deviated from (DH, 2002). The sponsor should ensure arrangements for audit are in place and takes place (DH, 2005).

Openness and transparency of audit results and the changes implemented should be routine. The publication of audits and provision of a centralised database of anonymised audit results create a huge learning resource for all. This leads to improved quality and greater financial benefits, a decrease in adverse events and generally a more happy, responsible and stress-free research workforce. As part of the process of information sharing and clarification, research forums, sub-groups or committees are, as discussed earlier, a valuable resource for researchers and those working in R&D departments. R&D departments should keep lists of such research networks, to which researchers, especially novices, may be referred.

## Research

Governance of research was long overdue and the research governance framework is a welcome and necessary tool. Questions have been raised about its application (Jones and Bamford, 2004): while some argue that more public debate is required (Soteriou, 2004), others state that, as a result of governance and the need for evidence-based practice, health professionals should be more ethically aware. Others believe that the public, through the media, is perceiving unethical conduct as a growing problem (Pettigrew, 2002), and that the care home sector poses particular issues because of its mixed public–private status (Reed et al, 2004).

There is an extremely thin line between research and audit. They probably have more commonalities than differences and, like research, audit has numerous definitions, each varying slightly. Reading several definitions of each would help the reader distinguish between the two (North Yorkshire Alliance R&D Unit, 2005). According to Wade (2005), each sets out with a question, which hopes to provide evidence to bring about change in practice and each will have a relevant and sound design and methodology in order to reach conclusions. It is also more likely that whatever is identified by audit will be implemented more readily than research findings. Hence, audit should be just as rigorously assessed and reviewed as research. Guidance, in relation to definitions and differences, is available (NICE, 2002; NHS R&D

Forum, 2006). It is always best to adhere to and maintain the highest standards. Therefore, if doubt exists, in the best interests of all concerned, the guidance and standards set by the research governance framework should be followed. Other factors, such as which projects should be referred to RECs (Wade, 2005) and how long data should be kept and which records should/could be destroyed, have also caused controversy and confusion within the R&D community.

In deciding whether a project requires REC approval, careful consideration should be given not so much to the distinction between research and audit, but to the nature of the project and its likely implications, according to Abbasi and Heath (2005). These authors believe that, because current definitions of audit and research are not informed by moral considerations, prior to publishing concerned editors should seek clarification so as to protect participants and prevent unethical practice in the future. Some R&D departments have implemented measures to suit their needs. For example, accepting studies that have been peer reviewed by universities or grant-giving bodies, instead of R&D peer review (Appleton and Caan, 2004). These and other concerns not clarified in the framework have since been addressed and several recommendations have been made by professional bodies and committees (BPS, 2004; Royal College of Nursing, 2004; BMA, 2005; NHS R&D Forum, 2006). It also behoves researchers to invoke change by being more proactive on RECs and R&D committees, and by keeping up to date with latest practice and new legislation (BPS, 2004).

Soon after the establishment of the Central Office for Research Ethics Committees (COREC), dissatisfaction with the ethics application process was reported in numerous articles in the professional media. Researchers still have reservations when going through this process, especially in relation to their chosen methodology, knowledge of the particular research participant group or lack of appreciation of the participant environment. Although there must be some collaborative studies between the NHS and social care, these reservations possibly arise more in the latter than the former, because of the lack of knowledge of social care science research methods.

Those involved in conducting and managing research should ensure that they are suitably qualified and/or have acquired the necessary experience and training for their role. Employers and R&D departments can assist here by including this in contracts, research agreements and handbooks for staff. Research assistants, new researchers and students should be given support, training and supervision commensurate to their needs (DH, 2005). It is good practice to appoint a named supervisor or mentor for the inexperienced researcher. In the author's experience, operating a mentoring system has proved to be extremely beneficial to the inexperienced researcher, the mentor, other researchers and the R&D department as a whole.

To assist organisations the DH makes recommendations, for example, on the use of a model clinical trials agreement (DH, 2004a); liaises with key stakeholders to produce information helpful to organisations in implementing the research governance framework accurately and efficiently; supports them with understanding their research governance duties (DH, 2005); and encourages and aids networks such as the R&D Forum and the Social Services Research Group.

Wherever research is conducted, there should be systems in place to ensure adherence to the research governance framework. If more than one organisation is involved, then the most suitable one should manage the framework measures. Research not undertaken on behalf of the NHS or social services is deemed to be private and is not the responsibility of NHS health and social care providers (DH, 2005). Apart from the above, the research organisation is primarily responsible for maintaining systems that ensure projects are conducted scientifically and ethically. Before a particular research project is undertaken it is important not only to gain informed consent from the participant, but also to inform all involved, whether in a caring or non-caring capacity (the organisation, formal or informal carers, next of kin or guardians), that the participant has been invited and has consented to take part. If there are objections, it would be wise to discuss this with the objector/s and the participant. If no consensus can be reached, it may be necessary to withdraw the participant, especially in the case of the elderly or young people.

The research governance framework (DH, 2005) states that any risks to participants, when the research is undertaken should be in proportion to the potential benefits and this must be very clearly explained to the REC or other ethics reviewer and the participant together with the arrangements for compensation in the event of non-negligent harm. It is a legal requirement to have insurance or indemnity for clinical trials involving medicines (DH, 2005). Where there are risks, it is deemed unethical to involve those who cannot or do not fully understand the implications, especially if there are no therapeutic benefits for them. Organisations who fund research have a duty to assess every proposal for scientific quality and value for money, the training and experience of researchers, the organisational and financial infrastructure behind them, and its experience with clinical trial management and compliance with good clinical practice and principles, especially in relation to trials on medicine.

## Conclusions and contemporary challenges for governance issues

The research governance framework is applicable to all research conducted by NHS-funded organisations and social services, whether clinical or non-clinical, involving human participants, their tissues, organs or data. Everyone, whether they are a researcher, funder, sponsor or formal carer, whether they work in R&D or an REC, whether they are a researcher's employer or in charge of an organisation where the research is being carried out, have roles, responsibilities and can be held accountable for their actions in relation to research. Hence, no employee in health and social care is immune from adhering to the research governance framework. Review committees should be less rigid and more aware of different methodologies, participant groups and their environments, especially when dealing with social care research applications. Ethical and moral issues should take precedence in reaching a decision as to whether the project should be categorised as research or audit. In summary, the salient components in maintaining and sustaining quality in research, according to the framework (DH, 2005), are respect for participants' dignity, rights, safety and well-being; valuing the diversity within society; personal and scientific integrity; leadership; honesty; accountability; openness; and clear and supportive management. The research governance framework (DH, 2005) provides most, if not all, of the answers as well as a sound structure and foundation for research. However, all the above is of very little value if research findings are not appropriately disseminated to provide the much needed evidence, capable of making a difference in all aspects of health and social care.

## References

Abbasi, K. and Heath, I. (2005) 'Ethics review of research and audit', *British Medical Journal*, vol 330, pp 431-2.

Alexander, J., Lee, S.-Y. and Bazzoli, G. (2003) 'Governance forms in health systems and health networks', *Health Care Management Review*, vol 28, no 3, pp 228-42.

Animals (Scientific Procedures) Act 1986 (Appropriate Methods of Humane Killing) Order 1996, London: The Stationery Office (www.opsi.gov.uk/si/si1996/Uksi_19963278_en_1.htm#fnf001).

Appleton, J. and Caan, W. (2004) 'Guidance on research governance', *Community Practitioner*, vol 77, no 8, pp 303-5.

BMA (British Medical Association) (2005) *Confidentiality as part of a bigger picture*, A discussion paper from the BMA (www.bma.org.uk).

BPS (British Psychological Society) (2000) *Code of conduct, ethical principles and guidelines*, Leicester: BPS Publications.

BPS (2004) *Good practice guidelines for the conduct of psychological research within the NHS*, British Psychological Society, Professional Practice Board, Division of Clinical Psychology, Research Ethics Practice Working Party After Training Strategy Group, Leicester: BPS Publications.

Bristol Royal Infirmary Inquiry, The (2001) *The inquiry into the management of care of children receiving complex heart surgery at the Bristol Royal Infirmary 1984-1995*, London: The Stationery Office (www.bristol-inquiry.org.uk/index.htm).

Data Protection Act 1998, London: The Stationery Office (www.opsi.gov.uk/ACTS/acts1998/19980029.htm).

DH (Department of Health) (1995) *The Patient's Charter and you – A Charter for England*, London: Patients Charter Unit, DH (www.pfc.org.uk/medical/pchrt-e1.htm#info-author).

DH (2000) *Research and development for a first class service*, London: DH.

DH (2001) *Research governance framework for health and social care* (1st edn), London: DH.

DH (2002) *Examples of good practice: Policy and guidance: Research and development*, London: DH (www.dh.gov.uk).

DH (2004a) *Research governance framework for health and social care: Implementation plan for social care*, London: DH.

DH (2004b) *NHS permission for R&D involving NHS patients*, London: DH.

DH (2005) *Research governance framework for health and social care* (2nd edn), London: DH.

Dolan, P., Woolham, J. and Manthorpe, J. (2004) 'Ethics review of social care research: Options appraisal and guidelines. Response of the ADSS to public consultation' (www.adss.org.uk).

Duffin, C. (2005) 'Testing research', *Nursing Standard*, vol 19, no 29, p 12.

Health and Social Care Act 2001, London: The Stationery Office (www.opsi.gov.uk/acts/acts2001/20010015.htm).

Health and Social Care (Community Health and Standards) Act 2003, London: The Stationery Office (www.opsi.gov.uk/acts/acts2003/20030043.htm).

Holmes, S. (2004) 'Is governance now inhibiting research?', *British Journal of Health Care Management*, vol 10, pp 305-9.

Human Rights Act 1998, London: The Stationery Office (www.opsi.gov.uk/acts/acts1998/19980042.htm).

Human Tissue Act 2004, London: The Stationery Office (www.opsi.gov.uk/acts/acts2004/20040030.htm).

Jamrozik, K. (2000) 'The case for a new system for oversight of research on human subjects', *Journal of Medical Ethics*, vol 26, pp 334-9.

Jamrozik, K. (2004) 'Research ethics paperwork: what is the plot we seem to have lost?', *British Medical Journal*, vol 329, pp 286-7.

Jones, A. and Bamford, B. (2004) 'The other face of research governance', *British Medical Journal*, vol 329, pp 280-2.

Mental Capacity Act 2005, London: The Stationery Office (www.opsi.gov.uk/acts/acts2005/20050009.htm).

NHS R&D (Research and Development) Forum (2006), 'Categorising research within the Research governance framework for health and social care', Version 2, July (www.rdforum.nhs.uk).

NICE (National Institute for Clinical Excellence) (2002) *Principles for best practice in audit*, Oxford: Radcliffe Medical Press Limited (www.nice.org.uk/pdf/BestPracticeClinicalAudit.pdf).

North Yorkshire Alliance R&D Unit (2005) *Research, audit or local service evaluation: A rose by any other name*, York: York Hospitals NHS Trust (www.northyorksresearch.nhs.uk).

Pettigrew, A. (2002) 'Ethical issues in health care research', *Radiography*, vol 8, pp 21-5.

Pierce, E. (2003) 'Research notes, how research and development centres and offices can assist you', *Nursing Standard*, vol 17, p 21.

RCN (Royal College of Nursing) (2004) *Research guidance for nurses*, London: Royal College of Nursing Research Society.

Reed, J., Cook, G. and Cook, M. (2004) 'Research governance issues in the care home sector', *NT Research*, vol 9, no 6, pp 430-9.

Royal Liverpool Children's Inquiry, The (2001) London: The Stationery Office (www.rlcinquiry.org.uk/download/index.htm).

Samanta, A. and Samanta, J. (2005) 'Research governance panacea or problem?', *Clinical Medicine*, vol 5, no 3, pp 235-9.

SDO News (2005) 'Researchers join forces to battle bureaucracy', Newsletter of the NHS Service Delivery and Organisation (SDO) R&D Programme, vol 8, no 1, London: NCCSDO.

Smith, P., Scott, J. and Pal, S. (2005) 'Awareness of research governance within a district general hospital', *Clinical Governance Bulletin*, vol 5, no 6, pp 2-3.

Soteriou, T. (2004) 'View from the research and development office', *British Medical Journal*, vol 329, pp 281-2.

Wade, D. (2005) 'Ethics, audit, and research: all shades of grey', *British Medical Journal*, vol 330, pp 468-71.

Wainwright, P. and Saunders, S. (2004) 'What are local issues? The problem of the local review of research', *Journal of Medical Ethics*, vol 30, pp 313-17.

WHO (World Health Organisation) (2004) *World report on knowledge for better health: Strengthening health systems*, Geneva: WHO Publications.

# FIVE

# Ethics and primary health care

*Charles Campion-Smith*

## Summary

The ethical aspects of everyday work in primary health care in the UK are discussed in this chapter. In this context, four main ethical concepts of beneficence, non-maleficence, autonomy and justice, described in Chapter Two, are reviewed within the context of primary health care. Issues such as the conflicting responsibilities for primary health professionals in their duty of care to an individual and to the greater community are discussed. The implications of evidence-based clinical care and the concept of clinical equipoise are considered, as well as issues of competence and consent. The uncertain and complex world of primary health care will be described as the setting for these issues and the allocation of restricted resources is reviewed. The need to take into account patients' views, beliefs and values as well as implications for teaching and research in primary care are discussed. Future challenges including the implications of the 2006 White Paper, *Our health, our care, our say*, are also considered.

## Introduction

While the ethical principles that underpin professional practice across the spectrum of health and social care work are largely consistent, the application of these principles has to reflect the particular context. Primary health care and the relationship that occurs between the patient or client and his or her professional attendants have some particular features.

In the UK and many other countries, general practice is the path by which people gain access to the range of health services to which they are entitled. While the degree to which a gatekeeping function is exercised varies, all general practitioners (GPs) have parallel obligations to individuals, communities and the state.

The key relationship between a professional and an individual may be nested within the relationship that the same professional has with other individual family members and the family as a whole. Additionally, GPs have knowledge of, and obligations to, the wider community; as a consequence the professional may have to balance competing considerations in the application of ethical principles.

The long-term or longitudinal relationship between a patient and professional, such as a family doctor, can foster the development of mutual trust, reinforced by shared experiences. Berger (1967) talks of the GP as the objective witness to the lives of patients or 'clerk to the records'.

Within this relationship the GP accompanies people as they make sense of what is happening to themselves – their bodies and sometimes their minds too. While colleagues working in hospital usually find the complaints from which the patients are suffering are more easily categorised into specific diseases, the disorders presenting in primary care, although real and bothersome, may not all represent a defined disease. How often will a GP hear patients describing their condition as "just not themselves", "not at all well" or "tired all the time"? Each of these complaints might represent a specific illness such as the onset of diabetes or thyroid disorder, but more often describes a state of unwellness that does not represent disease but may indicate distress which may originate from social or psychological discomfort or stress. As Heath (1995) writes, a key role of general practice is to patrol the border between the subjective experience of illness and disease and so protect people from medicalisation of the distresses of everyday life.

Primary care is a world of relative uncertainty, where critical judgements are made based on probabilities and where formulations are proposed provisionally. People's progress is observed over time and patients who do not follow the predicted path are re-evaluated. The professional, behaving ethically, is aware of both the benefits and harms of actions – such as referral to specialist services – and does not undertake these matters unthinkingly.

This discussion of ethics and primary care will use the concept of virtuous practice. Rachels (1999, p 173) defined virtue as "a trait of character, manifested in habitual action that is good for a person to have". More than simple knowledge is required as the arena is about the application and integration of this knowledge, as well as a demonstration of ethical professional standards. Virtues may be specific to a particular professional role; those appropriate for a primary care professional are considered.

In setting out the expectations that society has of professional behaviour, the aim is to provide a framework within which difficult decisions, taking into consideration both facts and values, can be made. Many would believe this to be the foundation that guides ethical practice.

## Three moral approaches

Three alternative, and often conflicting, approaches to ethical problems, namely utility, duty and virtue ethics (discussed earlier in Chapter Two), can be regarded as lenses through which an ethical question can be viewed. The application of these three moral approaches to primary care is now considered here.

Utility, or consequentialism, is an approach proposed by Jeremy Bentham and John Stuart Mill that regards the outcome or consequences of an action or decision as being paramount. All those affected are given equal weight. Utility can be summarised as aiming to achieve the greatest good for the greatest number. In health care this approach has impact when decisions about allocation of resources are being made. Primary care practitioners are often aware of conflict between their role as an advocate for an individual and the needs of the larger community.

Duty, or deontology, is a Kantian concept that states that all acts must be viewed as being morally significant in themselves, regardless of the consequences. The treatment of, and respect for, each individual is of greatest importance. This approach would oppose any act that involves withholding information from a patient even if justified as being in a patient's best interest. Any knowledge should be shared and there would be no place for the use of placebo interventions or even reassurance based on probability rather than firm fact. Duty-based theories encompass the contract between doctor and patient, the need to act to do good and to avoid harm, the recognition of patient autonomy and the fostering of trust and equity of provision.

Virtue ethics, derived from Aristotelian ideas, focus on the qualities, values and actions that we believe to be morally sound. Thomas Aquinas (1990) defined virtue as the habit or disposition of acting rightly according to reason. Virtue requires not only simple knowledge, but also the application and integration of this knowledge for a specific situation, a manifestation of ethical professional behaviour. This approach allows particular character traits to be valued for particular professions. The concept of the virtuous practitioner in primary care is discussed later in this chapter.

## Four ethical principles

Beauchamp and Childress (1989) have proposed that the four ethical principles of beneficence, non-maleficence, autonomy and justice, when used with attention to the context or scope of their application, provide a framework for clarifying thinking about ethical issues. Gillon (1994, 2003) has championed these ideas in the UK.

### Beneficence

To do good seems at first to be straightforward and not contentious but needs a clear view of what is in patients' best interest. Medicine is moving away from a paternalistic approach, where professionals make decisions on a patient's behalf with little acknowledgement of their beliefs, values or preferences. Preservation of someone's sense of control and identity is increasingly acknowledged to be sometimes as important as their physical health. In such a case support for a decision to refuse certain treatments which, viewed narrowly, might be seen to be of benefit, is appropriate and ethical. Here the balance between beneficence (to the physical state), non-maleficence (to the psychological state) and patient autonomy must be considered.

While no one would justify the withholding of requested care or attention to someone in genuine need, the same care and attention may be an inappropriate response to someone expressing distress from aspects of their life somatically. To collude with the medicalisation of such distress, while easier in the short term than challenging the patient's expectations and wishes, may well be harmful in rewarding dysfunctional behaviour rather than encouraging a more constructive approach to the problems. To challenge inappropriate requests for attention may be the considered response of a practitioner acting truly in a patient's best interest. Similarly, resisting demands for investigation or referral, while a likely cause of conflict or disagreement, may represent a thoughtful and ethically responsible approach. As Louise Terry points out in Chapter Two, providing benefit is not always possible.

Traditionally there has been an imbalance of power in the consultation; in the past a paternalistic approach has been the norm. While there are patients who still are happy to accept this approach (and in many ways this approach can be comfortable for the professional too) the ethically aware practitioner will be conscious of its benefits and harms, only using a paternalistic style when justified for a specific purpose.

To do good also requires that a professional remains up to date and appraised of current evidence for the effectiveness of different interventions and therapies. However, the professional will not let such evidence dictate the actions within an individual consultation, but will be aware of the limitations of the research and the applicability to the patient seeking advice. The task has been described as "fitting the square peg of clinical evidence into the round hole of patients' lives" (Freeman and Sweeney, 2001, p 1100). The findings from the research will be used to inform the discussion with the patient but never dictate the outcomes. The ethical practitioner will be aware of their preferences and will guard against allowing their personal views to distort the presentation of evidence for consideration. Edwards and Bastian (2001) discuss communication with patients about risk and benefit and suggest that professionals should demonstrate clinical equipoise, expressing no preference for a particular course of action. This approach is easier to achieve in areas where the balance of risk and benefit is fine, such as screening for prostate cancer or even primary prevention of cardiovascular disease in those at only moderate risk, but is more difficult to maintain when discussing issues such as the harms of smoking, where professional opinion is unequivocal.

Balint (1957) describes 'the drug the doctor' and Cassell (1991) talks of the healing relationship. In primary care, the ethical practitioner will be aware of the therapeutic power the relationship itself has and will use this powerful tool consciously and effectively. The ethical practitioner will find that being with a patient at times of difficulty or distress, such as loss or a diagnosis of a serious illness, brings benefit to patients, even though, seen objectively, the practitioner has done little. Similarly, care and time spent in thoughtful communication about important matters and particularly imparting bad news, can be a positively helpful act appreciated by patients.

## Non-maleficence

Patients should be protected from actual or potential harm whenever possible. The virtuous practitioner evaluates his own skills and knowledge realistically, undertaking only interventions for which he has the appropriate skills and knowledge. The virtuous practitioner recognises his personal limitations and potential sources of error (Klein, 2005), and will seek the advice of colleagues appropriately. Such a practitioner does not use unorthodox or unproven treatments except within a properly constituted trial and with the patient's fully informed consent.

The virtuous practitioner avoids hurt by empathetic and sensitive communication and will take into account and respect the values and beliefs of his patients. When errors occur the practitioner discusses these with the patient affected (unless considered that such discussion would be significantly harmful to the patient – for instance in raising unnecessary anxieties) and acts openly to minimise any adverse consequences.

The primary care practitioner is often closer to the patients and the realities of their lives than the hospital professional who may see patients briefly and is disconnected from their family and community. The GP has a role to protect his patient from the harms of well-intentioned therapeutic overenthusiasm and to make the patient clearly aware of the intended goals of the treatment proposed, be it a small chance of cure, remission or merely slight extension of life. The practitioner should remind patients of their right to discontinue a treatment that is making their remaining life a misery for little tangible benefit.

Practitioners will be aware that their support for and interest in a patient is a powerful therapeutic tool and that withdrawal of this approach can be an act of maleficence. In patients for whom cure is no longer possible and who are entering the terminal phase of their life, abandonment by professionals can be hurtful and harmful. The ethical practitioner will be aware that continuing commitment to these patients can help foster hope even in the most difficult circumstances (Buckley and Herth, 2004); such a practitioner will never say 'there is nothing more I can do'.

## Autonomy

Patients' rights to information about themselves and their condition should be respected and their views and beliefs heard and valued. This view may create difficulties when a patient chooses a different course from that recommended and indicated by clinical evidence, but the right to do so should be respected (Smith, 2002). However, if there are grounds to believe that someone's ability to make an appropriate decision is impaired, perhaps by the illness in question, the virtuous practitioner may decide to act in what is seen as the patient's best interest in order to receive the help needed. In the UK, sections 2 and 4 of the 1983 Mental Health Act enshrine this duty in the case of defined mental illnesses. Here is an instance of beneficence or non-maleficence overruling patient autonomy. As Louise Terry discusses in Chapter Two, appropriate balances have to be assessed with respect to autonomy when, for example, a patient would prefer to return home but the domestic environment has been judged to be unsuitable.

Autonomy becomes more problematic when choices are made on behalf of another such as a child or cognitively impaired relative. To what extent should a parent be able to make a decision that could prove harmful for their child? While at present parental decisions about choices such as the uptake of immunisations are accepted, more unusual cases, such as requests for prolongation of treatments thought to hold no prospect of recovery, or refusal to sanction life-saving surgery or transfusion, have been taken to the courts and parents' views overruled.

Autonomy is the principle that mainly impacts on issues of confidentiality and disclosure. A practitioner's first duty is to the patient. In most cases it is not contentious to disclose nothing to others without the patient's permission, either implicit, as in agreement to referral to another medical specialist, or explicit, where signed consent is obtained before disclosure to lawyers or insurance companies.

Research has shown that patients assume higher levels of confidentiality within general practices than is the case. In a questionnaire study, Wardman (2000) demonstrated that patients believed that access to their records by members of the practice's professional and administrative team was considerably more limited than is in fact usual practice. An ethical response to this finding might be for a practice to state openly who has access to the medical record.

Issues of confidentiality and autonomy become more complex when information gained from one patient has a major significance for others – to whom the professional may also owe a duty of care as patients of the same practice – or for the community at large. In such circumstances a practitioner must balance their duty to the individual with that to the wider community. Instances such as the patient who is a health professional, unwilling to disclose to employers that his ill health poses a risk of transmission of infection to patients, as well as the more familiar situation of the person with poorly controlled epilepsy who continues to drive, will present difficult dilemmas for the practitioner.

Practitioners can also be placed in a difficult situation when family members enquire about the health of relatives about whom they have concerns. While best care may be facilitated by open discussion of the problem by all involved or affected, there are times when the patient expressly forbids or blocks such a discussion and the practitioner may have to witness the confusion and distress of family members who cannot account for changed behaviour or attitude. Sometimes, highlighting the benefits of open discussion and exploring the fears that are leading to reluctance to discuss matters can be effective in bringing about more open dialogue to the benefit of both patient and carers.

Autonomy also encompasses issues of consent, which can only be valid if based on full disclosure of all the relevant information and the risks and benefits of the intervention. The concept of clinical equipoise includes the practitioner's duty to present information, free from personal bias or preference, in a way that allows an individual to make informed decisions. To assess someone's competence to make sense of such information may be important; too much information can overwhelm and be inimical to valid decision making.

When confronted with a seemingly illogical decision, the virtuous practitioner will explore with the patient the underlying reasons. When the decision is based on a fallacy or misconception correction may lead to a change of heart, but when strong underlying beliefs are uncovered the validity of the decision can be endorsed.

As well as consent to medical interventions, consent to the presence of health students in consultations must be specifically sought without penalty, actual or implied, for refusal. Similarly, research governance requires specific consent for participation in research with assurances that a decision not to take part will not influence the care received.

## Justice and equity

The Aristotelian principle suggests that a just system should ensure equals should be treated equally and unequals unequally. A procedural approach suggests that if the processes of allocation of goods and services are fair then this approach will contribute to a just outcome. Openness about the criteria on which decisions are made and their wide application across a system, such as the National Health Service (NHS), should help to avoid the perceived unfairness where access to certain drugs or procedures depends on where one lives – the so-called 'postcode lottery'.

Material principles of justice and equity allow decisions to be made as to whether resources should be distributed according to need, capacity to benefit, merit or rights. To distinguish between want and need is necessary and the professional may have to decide which needs should be met by health rather than by social, employment or housing services. There are also times when the professional may be aware of needs that a patient has not recognised. Capacity to benefit may be used to define eligibility criteria for procedures such as organ transplantation; decisions are made at a strategic level and the role of the GP is to explain and support the patient. Allocation on the basis of value judgements about relative merit or worth seems inherently unjust. For example, many smokers or overweight people feel they are discriminated against on these issues. Practitioners may, however, find it easier to help cooperative patients or those whose misfortunes arise through no fault of their own. Rights may be embodied in a contract or charter that includes entitlement to access to health care, confidentiality, respect and a response to concerns or complaints.

In many publicly funded health systems, such as the UK NHS, the primary care practitioner has a gatekeeper function, limiting the demand on the scarce and expensive secondary resources. The processes and material principles of justice will help the virtuous practitioner exercise this role cautiously. The foremost consideration should be clinical need rather than the patient's demand for preferment, acknowledging that the needs of the disadvantaged and less articulate or demanding patient may well be greater than those of those more insistent. Many would regard the role of an advocate for those less able to get the best from the system without such help as a key feature of virtuous practice.

Meanwhile in contrast to the UK NHS publicly funded primary health care system, in Chapter Two Louise Terry argues that justice suggests that patients with financial resources should contribute to the costs of social care.

The time and attention of practitioners themselves is another limited resource that will be allocated fairly in an ethical system. Communication with those from a different ethnic, social or cultural background from the practitioner, as well as those with impairment to speech or hearing, may be more difficult and the virtuous practitioner will take account of these factors.

## Virtuous professional practice

These four ethical principles may at times conflict. Critical judgement is required to choose which should take precedence. Gillon (2003) believes that respect for patient autonomy is a component of the other three and should be the overriding consideration. Gardiner (2003), a British GP, points out the limitations of these principles in the uncertain world of primary care where the emotional response of patient and professional must be taken into account. Gardiner (2003) proposes that the concept of professional virtue, which focuses on the character of the moral agent rather than the rightness of the action, may be useful in making such critical judgements. Gardiner suggests that a common benchmark is the question 'What would a good doctor do in this situation?'. The General Medical Council has also listed 'The duties of a doctor' (Box 5.1).

---

**Box 5.1:** The duties of a doctor (General Medical Council)

- Make the care of your patient your first concern;
- treat every patient politely and considerately;
- respect patients' dignity and privacy;
- listen to patients and respect their views;
- give patients information in a way that can be understood;
- respect the rights of patients to be fully involved in decisions about their care;
- keep your professional knowledge and skills up to date;
- recognise the limits of your professional competence;
- be honest and trustworthy;
- respect and protect confidential information;
- make sure that your personal beliefs do not prejudice your patients' care;
- act quickly to protect patients from risk if there is a good reason to believe that a practitioner or a colleague may not be fit to practise;
- avoid abusing your position as a doctor;
- work with colleagues in the ways that best serve patients' interests.

---

A more detailed description of the characteristics and actions of the excellent and unacceptable doctor is part of the current discussions about professional revalidation (GPC et al, 2002). More specifically for primary care, there have been a number of attempts to define what is meant by a 'good' or 'virtuous' GP. The Royal College of General Practitioners' report (1972), *The future general practitioner: Learning and teaching*, uses the behaviours and attributes expected and Toon's monographs on good general practice (1994) and the virtuous practitioner (1999) explore the topic further.

Virtuous practice requires the practitioner to take into account differing viewpoints and to recognise conflicts between the four ethical principles, while making critical judgements as to which to give greatest weight. In some situations, patient autonomy may permit courses of action such as refusal of recommended treatments to be taken that will be potentially or actually harmful. The situation becomes more complex when such decisions are made by one person on behalf of another such as a parent for their child. Should a parent's objections to surgery, blood transfusion or immunisation be respected, even if on balance the considered consequence is a greater risk of harm to the child?

Some believe that not only the behaviour but also the motivation determines ethical behaviour. Gardiner (2003) comments that the virtuous practitioner is driven by a deep desire to behave well and that this approach has a flexibility that can encourage innovative solutions while acknowledging that there will often be elements of pain or regret.

Rogers and Braunack-Mayer (2004) assert that the doctor giving excellent care, where such care is seen as a way to build a successful and financially rewarding practice, may be behaving in a less virtuous manner than another doctor whose motivation is less overtly businesslike and financial. However, there are undeniable benefits of financial reward, social status and job security that will have been a factor in the decision of many to join and remain in the profession. Nevertheless, there are possible factors as to why and how the professional driven primarily by financial or social success might be prompted to divide the limited resources according to benefits to the practitioner rather than according to the need of the patients seeking help.

Ethical practice includes demonstrating probity and professionalism in the use of professional status and in relationships with colleagues. While the virtuous practitioner should not undermine the standing of colleagues, there is also an obligation not to collude with unsafe or unsatisfactory practice. Clinical governance requirements include a responsibility to highlight such practice and 'whistle-blowing' is seen as a professional duty in such cases. These obligations are now made specific in the outline for professional revalidation (GPC et al, 2002).

## Future ethical challenges

Medical advances from prenatal diagnosis to the ability to sustain life longer bring dilemmas that will often be brought by patients and their families for discussion with primary care professionals who they know and trust; it is essential that these professionals are aware of the ethical considerations of such issues.

The 2006 UK White Paper *Our health, our care, our say* (Secretary of State for Health, 2006) is discussed in Chapter Seven, but also raises particular points for primary care. The move to bring services closer to patients' homes and to design the services around patients' needs and wishes is fully in line with the ethical principle of autonomy whereby the views and beliefs of patients should be heard and respected.

However, these changes mean professionals must be able to give appropriate information, without bias, to allow informed decisions to be made. The shift of services and resources to primary care offers opportunities for entrepreneurship – GP practices and others including the private sector have the opportunity to be both the commissioners and providers of care – but it is essential that there is absolute probity where there is a potential conflict between the priorities of successful business, spending of public money and service to patients. Most would welcome the White Paper's emphasis on better interprofessional working and the erosion of the barriers between health and social care, as discussed in Chapter Seven, but the necessary sharing of information raises challenges for the maintenance of confidentiality and the protection of data.

## Conclusion

Primary care practitioners are close to patients and their lives. Ethical challenges are present in many aspects of their practice and basic ethical principles, discussed more fully in Chapter Two, with an understanding of the concept of virtuous practice, can give a framework for addressing these issues but provide no easy answers. The nature of general practice in the UK is changing but strong ethical principles to underpin virtuous practice are important to assure the quality of the care delivered as the patients cared for become better informed and more consumerist in their approach to health care.

### References

Aquinas, T. (1990) *Summa theologica,* Latin original and English translation, Cambridge: Cambridge University Press.

Balint, M. (1957) *The doctor, his patient and the illness,* Tunbridge Wells: Pitman Medical Publishing Co.

Beauchamp, T. and Childress, J. (1989) *Principles of biomedical ethics* (3rd edn), New York, NY: Oxford University Press.

Berger, J. (1967) *A fortunate man,* London: Allen Lane.

Buckley, J. and Herth, K. (2004) 'Fostering hope in terminally ill patients', *Nursing Standard,* vol 19, no 10, pp 33–41.

Cassell, E. (1991) *The nature of suffering and the goals of medicine,* New York: Oxford University Press.

Edwards, A. and Bastian, H. (2001) 'Risk communication – making evidence part of patient choices', in A. Edwards and G. Elwyn (eds) *Evidence based patient choice: Inevitable or impossible,* Oxford: Oxford University Press, pp 144–60.

Freeman, A. and Sweeney, K. (2001) 'Why general practitioners do not implement evidence: a qualitative study', *British Medical Journal*, vol 323, p 1100.

Gardiner, P. (2003) 'A virtue ethics approach to moral dilemmas in medicine', *Journal of Medical Ethics*, vol 29, pp 297-302.

Gillon, R. (1994) 'Medical ethics: four principles plus attention to scope', *British Medical Journal*, vol 309, p 184.

Gillon, R. (2003) 'Ethics needs principles – four can encompass the rest – and respect for autonomy should be "first among equals"', *Journal of Medical Ethics*, vol 29, pp 307-12.

GPC (General Practitioner Committee), BMA (British Medical Association) and RCGP (Royal College of General Practitioners) (2002) *Good medical practice for general practitioners*, London: RCGP.

Heath, I. (1995) *The mystery of general practice*, London: Nuffield Provincial Hospitals Trust.

Klein, J. (2005) 'Five pitfalls in decisions about diagnosis and prescribing', *British Medical Journal*, vol 330, pp 781-3.

Rachels, J. (1999) *The elements of moral philosophy*, London: McGraw-Hill International.

RCGP (Royal College of General Practitioners) Working Party (1972) *The future general practitioner: Learning and teaching*, London: RCGP.

Rogers, W. and Braunack-Mayer, A. (2004) *Practical ethics for general practice*, Oxford: Oxford University Press.

Secretary of State for Health (2006) *Our health, our care, our say: A new direction for community services*, Cm 6737, Norwich: The Stationery Office.

Smith, R. (2002) 'The discomfort of patient power', *British Medical Journal*, vol 324, pp 497-8.

Toon, P. (1994) *What is good general practice?*, Occasional Paper 65, Exeter: Royal College of General Practitioners.

Toon, P. (1999) *Towards a philosophy of general practice: A study of the virtuous practitioner*, Occasional Paper 78, Exeter: Royal College of General Practitioners.

Wardman, L. (2000) 'Patients' knowledge and expectations of confidentiality in primary health care: a quantitative study', *British Journal of General Practice*, vol 50, pp 901-2.

# SIX

# Ethics and social care: political, organisational and interagency dimensions

*Colin Whittington and Margaret Whittington*

## Summary

This chapter describes examples of the values and ethical codes that aim to inform and govern practice in the overlapping domains of social care and social work in the UK. The provenance of these codes is considered. The history and nature of three broad streams of values that influence social care and social work are then described: 'traditional', 'emancipatory' and 'governance' values. The twin discussions of provenance and different value streams are used to argue that the codes manifest political and organisational dimensions as well as professional ones. The chapter then turns to a further dimension, interorganisational, and to a critical context for implementing values in social work and social care, namely interagency relationships. The three ethical themes of confidentiality, autonomy and justice, together with related practice issues, are then illustrated in the context of interagency relationships.

## Introduction

Ethics in social care and social work are typically expressed through professional ethical codes. Codes perform a number of functions (Banks, 2004), but stand formally as guides to expected conduct of practitioners. This purpose concentrates attention especially on the relationship of practitioner and service user. Yet consideration of ethical codes and of the values that influence such codes, reveals other contextual dimensions, each one carrying implications for the practitioner–service user relationship. The dimensions are political, organisational and interorganisational.

Our exploration seeks to draw out these different threads by citing examples of codes, considering their provenance and analysing values and ideas that influence codes. The exploration will help to show, first, that values and codes express political and organisational influences as well as professional ones; and second, that the provenance of some codes signify changing relationships between the professional service giver and, respectively, the service user and the state.

The chapter then turns to the interorganisational dimension and from historical and theoretical analysis to practice. Using case examples of three ethical themes, a critical context is illustrated for implementing values, namely interagency relationships in social care and health care.

## Social care and social work

The chapter refers both to 'social care' and to 'social care and social work' for the following reasons. The code of practice issued by the four UK national care councils (GSCC, 2002) applies the term 'social care' to embrace both social workers who number around 76,000 in England (Skills for Care, 2005) and the vastly greater numbers of other staff providing social care services. This usage reflects a wider, government-driven agenda directed to the collective 'modernisation' of a UK social care workforce of well over one million and of the services they provide (Secretary of State for Health, 1998).

Social care is, thus, both a set of services and the workforce providing those services. The dual convention is followed in speaking of the workforce collectively and, when necessary, of distinguishing between social work, as a distinct occupational group with a particular history and qualification and the wide variety of other social care staff.

## Professional values and ethical codes in social care and social work

Professional values are statements of belief about morally good or bad conduct (Clark, 2000). In social care and social work, ethics are typically expressed as descriptions or codes of required professional conduct, representing the active form of explicit, or sometimes implicit, values. Codes are illustrated below with summaries from three examples.

*UK code of practice for social care workers:* this code is issued from a common template by the four national regulators of social care and applies to all UK social care workers (GSCC, 2002). The code complements a code of employer responsibilities in the regulation of social care workers and lists the standards of professional conduct and practice required of staff in their work. For example, social care workers must:

- protect the rights and promote the interests of service users and carers, challenging discrimination;
- work to establish trust, respecting confidentiality;
- promote independence, respect users' rights to take risks but seek to protect users from harming themselves or others;
- uphold public trust;
- be accountable, work in partnership and improve the quality of one's practice.

*Code of ethics of the British Association of Social Workers (BASW):* the BASW code describes and prescribes five basic social work values and says how the values connect:

> Social work practice should both promote respect for *human dignity* and pursue *social justice*, through *service to humanity*, *integrity* and *competence*. (BASW, 2002, p 2; emphasis in original)

Each value is elaborated in a set of 'principles' and used to indicate required 'ethical practice' in relation to service users, the profession, workplace accountability and roles such as manager or educator. Ethical practice with service users includes promoting their interests and autonomy while protecting users and others, demonstrating cultural awareness, challenging oppressions and inequalities and observing confidentiality.

*The UK national occupational standards (NOS) for social work: Values and ethics statement of expectations:* the values and ethics statement of the social work NOS begins with a list that mingles expected skills and knowledge with desired ethical practice (Topss England, 2004). The list covers communication, advocacy, work with other professionals, professional knowledge and 'good practice'. The list also states separately the values to which social workers must subscribe, including honesty about role and powers, respect for diversity, putting service users first and empowering users, maintaining confidentiality and challenging discrimination.

## Reflections on the three 'codes'

A detailed reading of the GSCC, BASW and Topss documents shows differences in the way their authors approach the task and use terminology. However, it is evident, even from the brief summaries given above, that common domains and objectives are being addressed. All three examples amount to 'ethical codes' in the sense that they express required professional conduct based on implicit or explicit values. This chapter will not compare or critique the content of these codes, nor map their relationship to ethical theory since there are excellent tools for the task elsewhere (Clark, 2000; Banks, 2004; Beckett and Maynard, 2005). Instead, the discussion will consider briefly by whom and for whom the codes were produced.

BASW is a membership organisation and the code is produced by and for social workers. The model is characteristic for professions. The other two codes represent very different models for producing ethical rules and illustrate emerging political and professional dynamics.

The Council of the GSCC is not a body of like professionals. The members are appointed to reflect the diversity of social care stakeholders. The GSCC is funded by government and members are government appointees comprising a lay majority and lay chair. The GSCC code was compiled by wide stakeholder consultation and is not the product of a given professional or interest group. The standards, however, have the status of central criteria in the training, registration and de-registration of professionals in social work and social care.

NOS are statements of the competence needed in employment and are developed in social care and health by employer networks and other care interests supported by state-funded organisations. The standards are used as criteria in assessment for defined qualifications, as in the case of the social work NOS. The values and ethics statement of the social work NOS is based on consultations with service users and carers whose expectations are embodied in the statement and have become part of the occupational standards. This outcome means that service users and carers contribute criteria used in determining the competence of candidates for the degree in social work. In turn, the 'expectations' have been incorporated in occupational standards applicable to other care workers and their qualifications.

The GSCC and NOS codes illustrate two developments:

i) the voice of non-professional stakeholders, including service users and carers, given authority in the training and occupational requirements of professionals and in the governance of professional conduct;

ii) the deliberate hand of government in creating the structures and conditions under which that stakeholder authority may be established (Secretary of State for Health, 1998).

In 2005, legal protection was given to the title 'social worker' and celebrated as recognition as a profession. Yet the developments we have described are not the mark of a profession in the conventional mode (Higham, 2005). The hierarchy that has in some professions characterised the relationship between service user and service giver is altered. In addition, practitioner regulation is uncharacteristically 'external' and closely underwritten by government (Kingston, 2005).

In turning now to values and ideas that influence social care and social work and that, in varying degrees, gain expression in the codes, our chief source is social work.

## Streams of values

Founding influences on the values that shape contemporary social care can be seen in the precursors of modern schools of social work that appeared in the UK, mainland Europe and the US in the 1890s and early 1900s. These precursors were initiated by charitable movements, labour groups, movements of women and the churches, which were inspired by two broad sets of ideas: first, religious discourse, whose central position in the ethical development of individual casework represents a 'traditional' stream; and, second, the 'emancipatory' stream of a rapidly developing social reformism. A third and powerful influence crystallised later, as social work and social care became established as elements of organised service bureaucracies. This influence is referred to as the 'governance' stream to which the larger part of this discussion is devoted, as this stream is the least widely discussed of the three.

### Traditional stream

Social work developed in Europe and the US and social work values are grounded in assumptions about the individual and service to our fellow beings that strongly represent the influence in those regions of Christian or Judaeo–Christian discourse. Beckett and Maynard (2005) say that the other major religions of Islam and Buddhism have also influenced social work values but conclude that Christianity is the predominant religious source.

This source is famously expressed in *The casework relationship* written by a Roman Catholic priest (Biestek, 1961), which promotes the ethic of personal service rooted in recognition of the value, uniqueness and intrinsic worth of every individual who must be *respected*, a key idea, regardless of personal or social characteristic, history or behaviour. The source is also reflected, for example, in the founding role of Christian charities in social work in the UK and their continuing role in today's major independent agencies such as Barnardo's.

Reference to religion and to 'individualism' can take the discussion only so far in identifying the source of present-day professional ethics. To go further it is necessary to turn to the emancipatory stream.

## Emancipatory stream

The emancipatory stream in social work and social care is grounded in social reformism that explained the roots of poverty, crime and human distress in the way societies structured and distributed their wealth and opportunities. Measures to reform these causes of social injustice gained inspiration from Christian values, yet also reflected a quite different inspiration in the critical theories of Marx and his successors.

By the 1970s, the services and professions that had grown across the welfare state as part of the 1940s' postwar social settlement were under attack. In social work, a revived Marxism dismissed the person-focused social casework for critical docility towards an oppressive capitalist society. There were critiques of failing poverty programmes, continued homelessness, oppressive psychiatry and unequal criminal justice. These critiques broadened with the advent of feminism, anti-racism and gay rights movements, which challenged widespread institutionalised oppressions. The professionals who worked in the services did not escape but were castigated as being part of the problem.

Many social workers wished to be part of the solution. While their lobbying would have little direct influence on the broader structures of power and economic inequality, the injustice of racism, sexism and discrimination against homosexuality could be opposed in social work practice and declared in professional values. The subsequent dissent and debate gave voice to the ideas of equality, empowerment and anti-discrimination that have since become lodged in contemporary values and ethical codes of social work and social care as well as being extended to address the position of people with disabilities, older people and religious minorities. These ideas and concurrent growth of user movements, identity politics and consumerism have brought alliances with service users, recognition of the people who care for and support them, authentication of users' views of services and direct learning from their movements. The developments represent political processes and political outcomes.

## Governance stream

While left-radical critiques of welfare were raging at the end of the 1970s, economic recession and the arrival of the Thatcher government influenced by the free market economic theories and values of the 'new right' threw another critical spotlight on the welfare state. The critique claimed that services were inefficient, ill managed, lax in the use of public money and lacked accountability. The services were also professionally led, when they should be consumer-led and were unresponsive to individual need and choice that the market could best deliver.

The stance led to a programme of 'internal markets', tight controls on spending, targets, performance assessment, new national organisations for audit and inspection and injunctions both to compete and cooperate. This 'new managerialism' sought to supplant traditional bureaucratic administration and to challenge professional dominance.

By the arrival of a New Labour government in 1997, these methods and underlying ideas were firmly embedded across the public sector. New Labour revoked some of its predecessors' methods but has retained and extended others. Performance management and audit systems have been enlisted to monitor and support the ambitious 'modernisation' agenda, in which service partnership has a central role and is backed, variously, by exhortation, sanction and statutory duty (Whittington, 2003). Measures have been taken to strengthen public participation and accountability to stakeholders, while the goal of consumer choice has seen the return of market ideas.

Government investment in this agenda has been accompanied by growing recognition of the complex plurality of the systems that result and of the need to think of managing beyond organisations to 'whole systems'. A sense of the many risks that accompany these systems has also intensified with the accumulation of lapses in quality and serious failures (Secretary of State for Health, 1997; Secretary of State for Health and Secretary of State for the Home Department, 2003). The concept of 'governance' has emerged to capture the task, referring to a developing discourse of values and practices ranging from the service level of clinical and social care governance to corporate and extra-corporate levels. These values include probity, efficiency, partnership, the importance of managing risk, the right to high quality, effective services, involvement of service users and accountability to stakeholders, who include taxpayers, government and service users.

These values are articulated widely in statutory social care, the NHS and beyond. Many such values – for example, involvement of users, partnership, honesty, quality, risk management – are in harmony with traditional values of respect for people and the emancipatory values of justice and empowerment. In addition, social work and social care in the UK have typically gained their authority and functions from organisational employment and have built values of accountability to the employer into their ethical codes.

The earlier discussion of provenance found professional codes becoming the carriers of government and stakeholder influence. Reflection on governance prompts an extension of this analysis of the political dimension of codes. It is suggested that the general value of accountability, together with the convergence, described above, of some other governance values with traditional and emancipatory values, assist the percolation of political priorities and the managerial values that support such priorities, into the practice culture and codes of social care.

If governance were a discourse free of dispute, there would be little at issue, but the case is less simple. Governance is enacted in organisations that are often large and complex and whose mission of high quality service must be accomplished under challenging conditions that may include: contradictory government injunctions; tight financial limits; the scrutiny of a critical media; and imperfect governance techniques. Organisational interpretations of, for example, risk, targets or service priorities and the pursuit of auditable, standardised provision in social care sometimes conflict with traditional person-centred or emancipatory service values (Banks, 2004). This chapter now turns from the organisational to the interorganisational and directly to practice.

## Interagency context

The weight given to partnership in service modernisation has brought burgeoning interest in interprofessional relationships as different professions are grouped together increasingly into teams or newly integrated organisations. These changes do not dissolve all organisational boundaries, however, tending simultaneously to create new ones while leaving other structures unchanged. A plurality of organisations remains within a mixed economy of care that comprises not only an interprofessional arena for practice but an enduring interagency context as well.

This context has critical implications for implementing an ethical approach, as will be illustrated with vignettes relating to three ethical themes. The themes are based on disguised real cases from the perspective of local authority community care services (CCS) for older people.

---

**Confidentiality related to information sharing**

Mrs AX is an 84-year-old widow sharing a house with Mr BX, her 50-year-old son, who has long-term mental health problems and has had numerous admissions to psychiatric hospital, sometimes compulsorily, but is at present a voluntary in-patient. When at home, Mr BX is prescribed daily medication but takes this erratically and is generally hostile to mental health professionals. Mr BX has threatened Mrs AX physically and insists that both observe his restrictive rituals in the home. Mrs AX is nevertheless very protective towards her son and strongly believes her duty is to remain with her son.

*Ethical scenario*

Mr BX is due for discharge home soon and the social worker (entitled 'care manager' in many agencies) from the CCS seeks information. The social worker and Mrs AX, who is both a carer and potentially vulnerable relative, wish to participate in discharge planning and in assessment and management of any risks to Mrs AX. The social worker from the adult community mental health team (CMHT) recognises these needs as well as the potential gains to both service users of shared information. However, Mr BX, who has only recently begun to trust the CMHT worker, insists that discharge and treatment information should remain confidential.

*Interagency issues*

The two social workers share conceptions of the professional ethic of confidentiality and the sense of dilemma about Mr BX's injunction that information may not be disclosed. Both social workers also feel implicit pressure from their agency functions that focus their respective roles and define the 'service user'. To the CMHT worker, the service user is Mr BX, the 'adult with mental health problems'. To the CCS worker, whose agency function combines care of older people and a lead agency role for adult protection, the service user is Mrs AX.

---

Both social workers know that the position cannot be adequately resolved with reference to narrow interpretations of agency function or service user, nor to a professional vision of duty focused on an individual. The way forward has to be negotiated within a framework of interagency policies and methodology that specifically respond to a wider system view. A care programme approach (CPA) to Mr BX requires the involvement of his carer and other agencies, while reference to the multi-agency responsibility for adult protection means that the CMHT cannot respond in isolation to Mr BX's wish for confidentiality. The two workers must negotiate an approach with one another and with Mr BX and Mrs AX in this context.

## Autonomy related to risk and protection

Ms Z, 67, has a history of alcohol abuse and intermittent depression. Ms Z is periodically drunk at home, creating risk of fire and accidents. During these periods, Ms Z forgets to eat and take her medication and her flat becomes dirty but her fierce independence means that offers of regular domiciliary services are refused. Ms Z has little contact with family and is occasionally verbally abusive to neighbours, who complain. Ms Z is assessed as legally competent to make decisions.

### Ethical scenario

Members of the primary health care team (PHCT) are regular visitors. The GP (general practitioner) is called periodically by anxious neighbours and the district nurse visits to treat Ms Z's ulcerated leg. The PHCT are concerned about Ms Z's fragile health and the risks represented. PHCT members press the CCS to have Ms Z moved to 'high support housing' or residential care. The CCS share the concerns but Ms Z rejects the suggestion. Rather than put pressure on Ms Z, the CCS social worker proposes to seek alternatives that will help Ms Z retain some autonomy and choice.

### Interagency issues

The different approaches of the PHCT and CCS reflect layers of professional culture and agency function that influence priorities on autonomy. The PHCT's function is treatment and prevention of illness and they prioritise management of Ms Z's multiple conditions and risks. Team members tend to prescribe solutions as professional experts, to expect patient cooperation and to seek the support of other care agencies in achieving this outcome.

The functions of the CCS also prioritise risk, focusing not only on risks to safety but also to independence and applying these factors as criteria in the nationally prescribed framework for determining service eligibility. Both risks apply in this case and the scope for action on each is framed by the agency's obligation to provide help but to act only within its powers, which do not permit compulsion upon Ms Z. The CCS social workers practise a social model of care that values self-determination and uses counselling and trust to negotiate cooperation. Responding to risk means trying to reduce likely harms while recognising potential benefits.

Progress is found in the participation of a third agency. A jointly agreed plan between the CCS and the local mental health service for older people involves a joint risk assessment in consultation with the PHCT and additional supportive home visits to Ms Z by the community psychiatric nurse. The PHCT and neighbours are partly reassured and a measure of autonomy for Ms Z is, for the time being, preserved.

### Justice related to anti-discrimination

Mrs A, aged 82, becomes known to the CCS on referral of her husband who is terminally ill. The couple's long-term poverty is reflected in their dilapidated flat and few possessions. The couple have no family nor close friends. Mr A dies soon after referral and Mrs A is herself found to be physically unwell. Mrs A is also depressed and lacks motivation to care for herself. Mrs A is admitted to hospital where her physical condition improves with treatment, but Mrs A remains depressed and fearful about the future.

The social worker from the CCS attends the multidisciplinary ward meeting to discuss possible discharge plans. Hospital staff have prepared a report as a contribution to the assessment, proposing that the most supportive course would be to transfer Mrs A to residential care. The recommendation is based on Mrs A's long-term dependence on her husband, her low motivation, lack of confidence and poor home circumstances. These factors suggest limited potential for independent living and are emphasised in the report.

The social worker's previous knowledge of Mrs A and discussion with the GP who has known Mrs A for many years introduce a different perspective, which is that Mrs A had been led into a dependent role by her husband's forcefulness and violence. The oppression had contributed to her powerless self-image, low confidence and depression. Her poor motivation appears to stem from these factors and from the prospect of her dilapidated flat. The social worker proposes that they offer Mrs A a care plan of practical measures to improve the home environment and active support from herself and other services to assist a return home.

*Ethical scenario*

The social worker acknowledges reasons to doubt Mrs A's capacity for independence, but sees real social injustice in the existence that Mrs A had led with her husband and in her resignation that no other kind of life is possible for her. With the GP's support, the social worker argues that effort should be made to provide a final chance to Mrs A to regain some quality of life and independence. Failure to try would be to perpetuate the injustice. The social worker also perceives in the assessment practices operated jointly between the hospital and the local authority, potential for unintentional discrimination arising from a tendency to focus on older people's lost functions, inability and dependency.

*Interagency issues*

The assessment and care planning in this case bring together three agencies and three perspectives: the hospital, social services and primary care. The information on antecedents provided by the social worker and GP introduces a question of social justice that is not apparent from the perspective available to hospital-based assessors. Each perspective is articulated by professionals in consultation with Mrs A, but the perspectives differ because of different agency 'locations' and associated differences in perception of the service user. The possibility of unintentional discrimination is itself an interagency dynamic arising from the experience that social workers need hospital assessment reports that emphasise dependencies in order to meet local authority criteria for allocating care services. The case of Mrs A and the other cases described illustrate the importance of understanding the interagency context in implementing an ethical approach and demonstrate the positive difference that such understanding may make to the quality of service provided.

## Conclusions and contemporary challenges in ethics and social care

Our exploration suggests four contemporary challenges. The first challenge relates to the interorganisational dimension described above. The challenge is concerned with gaining recognition that collaborative practice is indispensably interagency as well as interprofessional. The challenge is also to develop ethical understanding and related research and training that address the complexities and pervasiveness of both interagency and interprofessional practice.

The second challenge relates to 'the political' and concerns the broad social justice objective of social care professions. A commitment to this objective has been a hallmark of national and international ethical statements of professional associations in social work, in which traditional and emancipatory values are invoked and a commitment declared to dispute oppressions and inequality with national governments (BASW, 2002). The limited ability of UK social work to be heard in national debates has been attributed to the slow pace of the professionalisation of social work, but that pace has accelerated under New Labour with the introduction of a new degree, protected title and a regulatory council. Yet social work's influence, as a distinctive lobby, has been simultaneously curtailed by social work's assimilation as an object of policy and regulation into the wider domain of social care and by the incorporation of social care codes and practice into government-endorsed systems of governance. The challenge for social work – and for social care more widely – is whether and in what ways the potential for independent social and political influence can be found and mobilised.

The third challenge connects the political with the organisational. The challenge arises in the intersection of values and is confronted when particular values, such as governance of risk or costs, are applied in ways that conflict with traditional and emancipatory values and when codes require this to be disputed (BASW, 2002; Topss England, 2004). The challenge is in how relatively powerless and largely organisationally dependent social care practitioners should respond and how practitioners may be supported.

Finally, the purpose universally professed for ethical codes is their benefit to the service user. This intention takes on new meaning as codes and wider systems of governance initiate and adapt to policies of user involvement. These policies were long sought and their progressiveness deserves credit. Their impact, however, must be measured in evidence of real change in the improved availability and quality of social care. There is a practical challenge to measure that change and an ethical obligation to do so.

## References

Banks, S. (2004) *Ethics, accountability and the social professions*, Basingstoke: Palgrave Macmillan.

BASW (British Association of Social Workers) (2002) *Code of ethics for social work*, Birmingham: BASW.

Beckett, C. and Maynard, A. (2005) *Values and ethics in social work*, London: Sage Publications.

Biestek, F. (1961) *The casework relationship*, London: Allen and Unwin.

Clark, C. (2000) *Social work ethics*, Houndmills, Basingstoke: Palgrave.

GSCC (General Social Care Council) (2002) *The code of practice for social care workers*, London: GSCC.

Higham, P. (2005) 'What is important about social work and social care?', *SSRG (Social Services Research Group) Newsletter*, July.

Kingston, R. (2005) 'The regulation of the social care workforce as defined by the Care Standards Act 2000', Research paper, unpublished.

Secretary of State for Health (1997) *The New NHS: Modern, dependable*, Cm 3807, London: The Stationery Office.

Secretary of State for Health (1998) *Modernising social services*, Cm 4169, London: The Stationery Office.

Secretary of State for Health and Secretary of State for the Home Department (2003) *The Victoria Climbié Inquiry: Report of an Inquiry by Lord Laming*, London: The Stationery Office.

Skills for Care (2005) *The state of the social care workforce 2004: Second annual report (summary)*, Leeds: Skills for Care.

Topss England (2004) *The national occupational standards for social work* (retrieved 16 September 2005 from www.topssengland.net/files/SW%20NOS%20doc%20pdf%20files%20edition%20Apr04.pdf).

Whittington, C. (2003) 'Collaboration and partnership in context', in J. Weinstein, C. Whittington and T. Leiba (eds) *Collaboration in social work practice*, London: Jessica Kingsley, pp 13-38.

# SEVEN

# Ethics and interprofessional care

*Audrey Leathard*

## Summary

Ethics and interprofessional care are briefly defined to clarify a fourfold pathway for analysis. *Beneficence:* for whose good and who benefits from working together for health and social care? *Confidentiality:* how far can trust and private information be upheld for service users, across the differing administrative and professional boundaries? *Accountability:* to what extent can interprofessional work be held accountable to audit and regulation, to the rules of professional bodies, to management targets as well as to service users? *Collaborative governance:* as governance increasingly cuts across the public, private and voluntary sectors, how far can partnership working promote user involvement? One challenge for interprofessional care is to ensure that service users gain from these ongoing developments in policy and provision that requires effective evaluation.

## Definitions

*Interprofessional care* involves a range of terms and meanings that, overall, denote working together for service users across health and social care. However, increasingly the interprofessional field has extended to include, for example, children's services and housing as well as the voluntary and private sectors. The three main interprofessional arenas cover: (a) *conceptual issues* such as multiprofessional, interdisciplinary and multidisciplinary working; (b) *the process-based approach* such as team working, mergers, partnership working, joint working, collaboration and integration; and (c) *the agency-based arena* that includes interagency working, health alliances, consortiums, forums, federations and locality groups (Leathard, 2003, p 6).

Ethics relates to moral principles and codes that pertain to the distinction between right and wrong in relation to actions, volitions or to the character of responsible beings. Banks (2004, pp 3-4) makes a further distinction between ethics and professional ethics that covers such issues as the norms and standards of behaviour of members of specific occupational groups; of their sets of accepted values, ethical principles and rules of professional conduct; as well as their first professional loyalty that lies with the client/patient/service user.

From this background, four ethical principles are now applied to the place of interprofessional care: beneficence, confidentiality, accountability and collaborative governance. These principles have been selected as of particular relevance to the field of interprofessional work.

## Beneficence

Beneficence underlines the principle that the well-being of the individual ought to be promoted. In a similar sphere, the principle of non-maleficence indicates one ought to do no harm. Beneficence is therefore concerned with promoting benefit that immediately raises the question as to what is to count as benefit, for whom, by whom and who should make the assessment? As Singleton and McLaren (1995, p 45) set out, the duty of beneficence is an imperfect duty where individuals can consult their own inclinations about who shall benefit. Nevertheless, the promotion of the well-being of the individual remains at the centre of health and social care.

In turning to the field of interprofessional care, the place of beneficence encounters an immediate stumbling block: the relative lack of evaluation as to who actually benefits from working together across the health and social services. Some examples are now set out as to where studies have shown that benefits have occurred or faced setbacks.

1. One of the most positive outcomes for service users, with regard to collaboration between health and social care, is reflected in Turner and Balloch's (2001) study on the Wiltshire and Swindon Users' Network. From 1993, the main purpose has been to provide a support network for service users; to build up a membership organisation of service users to become involved in the planning, delivery and evaluation of services; to enable direct links between service users and the social services department; and to involve users in the programme based on a community development approach. Financial support was variously secured by special funds for user-controlled research from the Wiltshire County Council, the local health authority and the

Independent Living Fund. The Joseph Rowntree Foundation also contributed funds to undertake a user-controlled 'Best Value' survey for Wiltshire's direct payment scheme.

The outcome of the Wiltshire Users' Network has been upheld as a model for user involvement in evaluating services. In terms of who benefits most, user groups are, however, concerned with the particular needs of the better represented groups such as people with disabilities and older people, those with learning difficulties, mental health service users and, in some areas, young people in care.

2. Meanwhile, a two-year evaluation of integrated working between the health and social services for the joint commissioning and provision of mental health services in Somerset has shown that the process was less than seamless, while the benefits to users were not significant. Although structural innovation with good political support and some high quality management had been evident, together with initiatives to further user involvement and networking among unpaid carers, little shift of power had taken place towards users (Peck et al, 2002).

3. In contrast, from the National Primary Care Research and Development Centre at the University of Manchester, Glendinning and Rummery (2003, pp 186-99) have been assessing how primary care groups/trusts have responded to the emerging collaborative agenda with social services, more particularly in developing services for older people. The benefits have shown that interprofessional and interagency barriers are starting to break down between the centrally structured National Health Service (NHS) primary health care services and the elected local authority social services. However, the benefits differ between the primary care trust boards that tend to consult their professional colleagues rather than the older people themselves. In contrast, the values and perspectives of the social services professionals indicate a willingness to listen to older people, as well as to extend the benefits to this client group to enable involvement with planning, monitoring and reviewing service developments.

4. *Mergers:* a more negative example of beneficence has revealed, from a substantial study undertaken by the London School of Hygiene and Tropical Medicine (Fulop et al, 2002), that mergers may not necessarily be advantageous, serviceable or beneficial. Throughout 1998-99, mergers covering acute hospitals, mental health services and community provision showed that improvements for patients were delayed by at least 18 months, failed to deliver promised savings and did little to

improve staff recruitment or retention. From the setting of nine trusts and four case studies on trusts in London, there was no clear evidence that any savings had been reinvested into services nor even achieved, while savings on management costs took some two years. The only benefits to emerge were the bigger pool of professional staff that allowed larger teams of clinical specialists, training improvements and less fragmentation in mental health care. The time factor in perceiving benefits can be lengthy without any clear pathway as to who really gains from such mergers.

5. *Care trusts:* a more recent example of interprofessional and interagency developments through care trusts has, however, shown positive benefits for the future. Care trusts were first announced in *The NHS Plan* (Secretary of State for Health, 2000) to improve continuity and integration between the centrally run health services and the locally run elected social services, although both come under the overall direction of the Department of Health. From April 2002, focused on the needs of patients and users, care trusts started to be set up under joint agreement to provide integrated health and social services to the local community.

So who has benefited so far? By 2005, some eight care trusts had been formed with more intended to follow. An early review by Glasby and Peck (2004) has shown that health and social care staff are trying to enable better outcomes for service users from the resources available. However, while the government is seeking to improve collaboration between the health and social services, benefits only occur when local relationships are already good and the services have been moving forward together in the first place. Nevertheless, where agencies work together, local services can be improved for users and the more efficient use of resources can be made through pooled budgets.

Already by 2005, more positive outcomes can be seen, for example, with the Witham, Braintree and Halstead Care Trust which now commissions and provides health care to the community and social care, delegated by the local authority, for older people and other groups. Service duplication has significantly lessened, while better, more accessible services have benefited general practitioners (GPs), patients and users overall (Shepherd, 2005). Interprofessional care has therefore enabled benefits, through working together across health and social care, but more needs to be achieved to extend beneficence in this field. As Louise Terry points out in Chapter Two, under ethical theories and principles, beneficence and non-maleficence are often seen as two sides of the same coin. However, while a positive obligation not to harm exists, providing benefit is not always possible.

## Confidentiality

Confidentiality concerns the trust, confidence and reliance that patients and service users can expect from professionals where private and sensitive information is involved. Confidentiality is therefore a moral, professional, contractual and legal duty. However, as Singleton and McLaren (1995, pp 103-6) set out, exceptions to the necessity to maintain confidentiality include: with the individual's consent and public interest, under court orders or statutory requirements. Further, enshrined in the professional codes of conduct for nursing, midwifery, health visiting and medicine is the acknowledgement that information given by individuals to professionals should be held in strict confidence. However, the British Medical Association does recognise that exceptions in the duty of confidentiality can arise.

### Confidentiality applied to interprofessional care

In working across health and social care, the place of securing or even sharing confidential information can be problematic. The outlook of distinct professional groups, based on a specific set of ideals and ethical principles, may then have to be reviewed as professional roles become interchangeable, especially across community work. Where interprofessional and interagency working are increasingly linked together, so different agencies develop a unified strategic approach to address specific problems. Further professionals, with formerly distinct roles, may coordinate their work in order to meet the needs of service users more effectively, particularly in teams working for older people. However, professionally defined standards tend to be relatively general as practitioners, working in a wide range of settings which include the public, private and voluntary sectors, need some freedom to interpret, address and apply the ethical principle of confidentiality to particular cases.

The upshot is that the relationship between nurse and patient or between doctor and patient is 'special' and subject to codes of conduct (Rumbold, 2003, p 151). However, the place of interprofessional care opens up wider relationships that may challenge the more manageable ethical format for health care professionals. Further, some information across health and social care is not necessarily confidential which then raises the question as to how far and whether the patients' and service users' right to confidentiality is absolute, together with what type of information is relevant in this context.

A collaborative approach to health care ethics is essential, according to Kath Melia (2004, p 133), to put patients first and to respect their rights. The ethical challenge is to incorporate social care appropriately with respect to confidentiality. With the blurring of professional and practitioner boundaries, with partnership and team working developments moving apace, interprofessional values and procedures could appear to threaten the distinct professional groups with their own set of guiding ideals, ethical principles and rules. However, from the literature on interprofessional working, together with an account of the multiagency partnerships between the police, probation services, social services, health, education and the voluntary sector, Banks (2004, p 131) concludes that interprofessional working has become a generally accepted aim of central and local government.

The main justification has been that, where matters work well, the results have shown improved services for users; a reduction in service overlap provided by different agencies; greater consistency and continuity of services; as well as better communication and information sharing between professionals in order to provide a more streamlined service. Provided the interchangeability of roles and tasks is carefully considered, interprofessional working does not necessarily pose a threat to the place of separate professions and their distinct code of ethics (Banks, 2004, p 147).

With respect to confidentiality, one way forward may be to establish between the professional groups, sectors and organisations involved, an agreed code of interprofessional ethics that reflects the needs of practitioner groups, patients and service users across health and social care. Such a development could even consider a new body to address these matters. Alternatively, the UK Centre for the Advancement of Interprofessional Education (CAIPE) might be another appropriate organisation to involve in this arena. However, as interprofessional work continues to stretch across the voluntary and private sectors, so matters become more complex. Meanwhile, the arena could be overtaken by the increasing development of the new accountability with the imposition of procedures and targets for the professions involved.

## Accountability

To be accountable across health and social care provision concerns the requirement for the services and personnel involved to be able to provide an account, both financial and professional, of what has or has not been undertaken on behalf of the patients and service users. Practitioners and administrative staff are accountable to employers and management; practitioners and their employers are also accountable to the public for the effectiveness of the services provided. To enable professional and public accountability to be judged and reviewed, ever more measures have been introduced by employers to assess contracts, quality standards and complaints procedures. In part, the purpose seeks to respond to service users' demands for more effective services that take account of user views and participation in decision making.

## New accountability

The new accountability places an increasing focus on detailed procedures for undertaking tasks and setting predefined targets; to meet the requirement for quantifiable work outputs, with greater demands from internal and external regulation and audit. The purpose of the new accountability is to enable professionals to achieve more effective working and to improve practice. However, the overall outcome may pose a threat to professional ethics where the development of ever more detailed procedures, predefined targets and work outcomes appear to restrict the exercise of professional discretion and autonomy (Banks, 2004, p 149).

In contrast to the complexity of accountability across health and social care, interprofessional working is not necessarily accountable on the basis of a joint format although accountable in the separate spheres of health and social services where relevant. In terms of accountability, different sectors work to different financial agendas. Local authority social services departments are accountable to the chairs and councillors of various local committees and, through local elections, democratically answerable to the local voters. Meanwhile, the health services are directly accountable to the centralised structure of the NHS under the Department of Health which also holds social services centrally accountable. The continuing structural divide between health and social services provides both an ethical and contemporary challenge for interprofessional accountability.

Furthermore the private sector organisations, ever more drawn into partnerships with public and voluntary agencies, are legally and in practice responsible to their shareholders. The arena of partnership working and accountability can therefore be financially complex. Health and social care agencies have different budgetary and planning cycles, lines of accountability and levels of discretion accorded to frontline workers. The need for clear lines of management and accountability with regard to partnership agencies are therefore likely to be a sensitive area of interprofessional working (Balloch and Taylor, 2001, pp 22, 123).

## New ethical challenges for accountability in the 21st century

By July 2005, the Foundation Trust Network represented all 32 foundations trusts (along with 10 aspirant trusts). The Network wanted to see a freeing up of the foundation trust model to enable the provision of primary care services, access to primary care funding as well as to deliver the management of long-term conditions (Mooney, 2005).

The key distinction between the NHS hospital trusts and foundation trusts is local autonomy. Foundation trusts are intended to become more accountable and responsive to their local communities, run by locally elected boards with hospital staff and primary care trust representatives, together with more financial freedom and incentives to be entrepreneurial, innovative and free of regulation from central government (Leathard, 2005, pp 145-6). Foundation trusts have in theory greater freedom over pay, recruitment, financial control and tailoring services to meet local needs.

However, among the Foundation Trust Network's future recommendations are: to form partnerships with primary care services; to develop different types of care for patients with long-term conditions; to increase the freedom to borrow from commercial tenders; and to deliver services across the community, including social carer and community regeneration (Mooney, 2005). Just where accountability comes in, to whom, by whom and for whom, is not clear nor is the relationship with local authorities on social care provision.

Accountability could be further challenged by the opening up of new independent providers at the margins of primary care (McGauran, 2005, p 14). Meanwhile, 'partnerships' between the NHS, local authorities and other bodies are proliferating. The main issues concern how interprofessional and interagency working can deliver better, more seamless services to users. However, the proper accountability of interprofessional working also matters because, as Campbell (2004) discusses, the public and those affected by the decisions taken have a right to know. Meanwhile, the key factors for accountability cover the responsibility for the effective and efficient use of public services; who is taking decisions and how the public can influence the process; the responsibility for wrongful outcomes; and the need for accessible forms of redress.

To make partnerships more accountable, clarity is needed over the primary purpose involved (whether to make decisions or to act as a consultation forum), while the role of each partner should be clear and accountable, particularly with respect to control over or access to budgets. Further, partnerships with decision-making powers should be explicit about how they are accountable to their members, to stakeholders outside the partnership including funding bodies, as well as to service users and the public. However, Campbell (2004) concludes that despite an ever increasing number of partnerships between the NHS and local authorities, accountability is often minimal.

## Accountability and ethical challenges

While retaining existing employment regulations, the integrated health and social care staff under a single care trust management structure has required appropriate professional accountability and supervision arrangements. Linked to accountability has therefore been the necessity to identify professional leads within the integrated teams. Further, a key ethical lesson has shown the need to enable local collectiveness across interprofessional agencies so that working practices drive towards a common purpose (Glasby and Peck, 2004).

An ethical challenge to be resolved concerns representation and accountability. In looking at partnerships and power in community regeneration, Mayo and Taylor (2001, p 48) have found their community studies reflect differing needs and divisions of 'race', ethnicity, gender, disability, age and social class among other factors. How to represent these varying complex interests to the relevant community boards presents one problem, as does the need to establish effective channels of accountability where the process for monitoring and accounting is complex.

Overall, key questions for accountability across interprofessional care have to address: who undertakes the exercise? For whom and to what extent is the outcome effective for the future of agencies and sectors working together for the benefit of patients and service users?

## Collaborative governance

Governance is concerned with the framing, orientation and implementation of policies (Daly, 2003). From 1997, under the New Labour programme for the UK, public participation initiatives have shifted towards a more collaborative form of governance that is reflected in the language of policy documents. The approaches to policy implementation have increasingly been based on interprofessional, interagency, partnership working and user involvement that have led to a significant basis for evaluation as well as to pooled budgets and new forms of 'networked' and collaborative governance (Taylor and Balloch, 2005, p 4).

As a result, a greater emphasis is being placed on public participation in decision making, local involvement, alongside new forms of engagement between public sector agencies, consumers, users and communities. In this light, collaborative governance can therefore be seen as a positive arena to encourage interprofessional working.

However, as Newman et al (2004) point out, new forms of governance do not necessarily displace the old but can often interact 'uncomfortably'. The contentions occur in the changing relationships between central and local governance as well as between representative and participative democracy. In this context, moves towards collaborative governance may encounter conflict and constraints.

A further challenge to collaborative governance comes with the involvement of the private sector, more particularly for primary care. In June 2005, the Department of Health's plans were set out in *Creating a patient-led NHS: Delivering the NHS improvement plan* (DH, 2005). For primary care trusts, 'choice menus' are to be boosted by the inclusion of foundation trusts and independent treatment centres from April 2006. Patient choice is intended to be increased further by making a significant proportion of the existing private health care capacity available to NHS patients.

Meanwhile, independent providers are also required to meet NHS standards, to be able to provide care at the NHS tariff and to guarantee availability. In this context no mention has been made, so far, of collaborative governance through working together with social care. However, independent providers are to be added to the list of individual primary care trusts. One aspect of collaborative governance is intended through primary care trusts joining together to make contracting with providers more efficient. In this context, the development of 'partnerships' can be seen moving forward significantly, so that more public–private partnerships can be expected in the future (*Health Matters*, 2005, p 2).

Closer financial collaboration between the NHS and social care services has already been brought into section 31 of the 1999 Health Act that enabled pooled budgets by the partner organisations, as well as the commissioning of an integrated range of health and social care services. The flexibilities required for the establishment of new governance arrangements have also provided a framework for partnership working (Glasby and Peck, 2004, pp 1-5). Significantly, the development of care trusts has forced localities to address human resources and governance arrangements (Giles, 2004, p 81) together with the integration of financial and structural systems between the NHS centralised health care service and local government social care.

Collaborative governance has therefore played an increasingly significant part in the context of health and social care provision as one reflection of the present emphasis on public participation initiatives. As Newman et al (2004) discuss, the role of the state is moving from 'governing' through direct forms of control (hierarchical governance) to that of collaborative governance that involves different levels of decision making across a wide range of networks in the public, private and voluntary sectors. Interprofessional, interagency and partnership working have also all played a part towards agencies working together with the community involvement of service users. A significant move has therefore taken place towards a more collaborative style of governance in order to encourage active citizenship, to overcome social exclusion and to promote public participation and consultation alongside public involvement in decision making.

## Partnership working

Closely linked to collaborative governance is partnership working. The issue of how to govern and manage partnership working appropriately has increasingly risen to near the top of the public sector management agenda. With the expanding integration of health and social care agencies, by 2006 about 5,500 partnerships had been formed in the UK that controlled some £4 billion of public expenditure. However, for service users, further integration has often resulted in a lack of clarity about who is responsible. Indeed, as the Audit Commission (2005) has pointed out, there should be clarity in partnerships, spelt out in comprehensive agreements between partners. However, according to the Audit Commission's (2005) findings, most public bodies do not have such agreements for some of their partnerships. Furthermore, a clearer focus on accountability and evaluation is needed with regard to partnership involvement, resource implications and management (Strachan, 2006). So working together in partnerships has much to offer in order to further interprofessional care, which is strongly supported and furthered by the work of CAIPE. However, the ethical challenge is to ensure that partnerships benefit users as well as being effectively governed and accountable to both the relevant public bodies and to the general public.

## A new direction for community services

Closely linked to partnership working are the Health Secretary's proposals contained in the January 2006 White Paper *Our health, our care, our say* (Secretary of State for Health, 2006). The White Paper sets out the government's vision to provide more effective health and social care services outside hospitals, which significantly calls for joint commissioning of services between primary care trusts and local authorities.

Five clear areas for change are identified:

- personalised care to be driven by better access and more funding to follow the patient, while NHS walk-in centres are also to be expanded;
- services are to be brought closer to people's homes through investment in community hospitals;
- increased choice is to be underpinned by a direct payment or care budget for people to pay for their own home help or residential care;
- prevention of illness is to be targeted through the establishment of more health care teams to deliver better care across institutional boundaries;
- and, significantly for interprofessional care, better coordination between local councils and the NHS, which is to be a key goal to be led by the Department of Health's director of adult care services. A vital part of the vision is to improve the way information is shared between social services and health care providers.

Among the concerns at the heart of the proposals are, significantly for interprofessional care, that services will be integrated, built around the needs of individuals and not service providers, in order to promote independence and choice. The overall intention is to focus on partnership working, joint planning, prevention, budget setting and commissioning, monitored by a performance framework. Of significance across the proposals is to note that partnership working between health and social care is given a significantly high priority whereby health and social care services will have to work more closely together to plan services and budgets jointly (*Health Service Journal*, 2006). Alongside the implications for interprofessional work in the 2006 White Paper, Dr Campion-Smith also looks at the issues raised for primary health care in Chapter Five.

## Conclusions and contemporary challenges

In reviewing ethics in the context of beneficence, confidentiality, accountability and collaborative governance, positive developments have taken place to further the work of interprofessional care, but the need for ongoing evaluation remains a key factor. Through the Secretary of State's (2006) new direction for community services on health and social care working together in partnership, an increasing emphasis has been placed on service integration. By August 2005, the Department of Health has also been considering imposing a legal duty on rationalised primary care trusts and local authority social services to work together to improve adult care and to cut management costs. Meanwhile the government is rigorously examining reconfiguration proposals that would see the number of primary care trusts reduced significantly by over one half to 131 (Martin, 2006), to improve coterminosity with local authority social services departments. A further market upheaval is expected with the opening up of primary care to the private sector (McGauran, 2005, p 12). The implications for ethics and interprofessional care as well as for the patients and users involved remain to be seen but all of which are likely to set major contemporary challenges for the future.

### References

Audit Commission (2005) *Governing partnerships: Bridging the accountability gap*, London: Audit Commission.

Balloch, S. and Taylor, M. (2001) *Partnership working: Policy and practice*, Bristol: The Policy Press.

Banks, S. (2004) *Ethics, accountability and the social professions*, Basingstoke: Palgrave Macmillan.

Campbell, F. (2004) 'Alliances or dalliances?', *Health Matters*, issue 55, Spring, pp 16-17.

Daly, M. (2003) 'Governance and social policy', *Journal of Social Policy*, vol 32, part 1, pp 113-28.

DH (Department of Health) (2005) *Creating a patient-led NHS: Delivering the NHS improvement plan*, London: DH.

Fulop, N., Protopsaltis, G., Hutchings, A., King, A., Allen, P., Normand, C. and Walters, R. (2002) 'Process and impact of mergers of NHS trusts: multi-centre case study and management cost analysis', *British Medical Journal*, vol 325, no 7358, p 246.

Giles, S. (2004) 'Care trusts: a positive option for service improvement', in J. Glasby and E. Peck (eds) *Care trusts: Partnership working in action*, Abingdon: Radcliffe Medical Press, pp 77-82.

Glasby, J. and Peck, E. (2004) *Care trusts: Partnership working in action*, Abingdon: Radcliffe Medical Press.

Glendinning, C. and Rummery, K. (2003) 'Collaboration between primary health care and social care – from policy to practice in developing services for older people', in A. Leathard (ed) *Interprofessional collaboration: From policy to practice in health and social care*, London: Brunner Routledge, pp 186-99.

*Health Matters* (2005) 'Editorial', issue 60, Summer, p 2.

*Health Service Journal* (2006) 'Bridging the care divide', vol 116, no 6003, 27 April, p 7.

Leathard, A. (ed) (2003) *Interprofessional collaboration: From policy to practice in health and social care*, London: Brunner Routledge.

Leathard, A. (2005) 'Evaluating interagency working in health and social care: politics, policies and outcomes for service users', in D. Taylor and S. Balloch (eds) *The politics of evaluation: Participation and policy implementation*, Bristol: The Policy Press, pp 135-51.

McGauran, M. (2005) 'Market upheaval imminent', *Health Service Journal*, vol 115, no 5964, p 12.

Martin, D. (2006) 'Resubmitted plans face DoH scrutiny', *Health Service Journal*, vol 116, no 6003, 27 April, p. 9

Mayo, A. and Taylor, M. (2001) 'Partnerships and power in community regeneration', in S. Balloch and M. Taylor (eds) *Partnership working: Policy and practice*, Bristol: The Policy Press, pp 39-56.

Melia, K. (2004) *Health care ethics*, London: Sage Publications.

Mooney, H. (2005) '"Boutique" model mooted', *Health Service Journal*, vol 115, no 5963, p 6.

Newman, J., Barnes, M., Sullivan, H. and Knops, A. (2004) 'Public participation and collaborative governance', *Journal of Social Policy*, vol 33, part 2, April, pp 203-23.

Peck, E., Gulliver, P. and Towell, D. (2002) *Modernising partnerships: An evaluation of Somerset's innovations in the commissioning and organisation of mental health services: Final report*, London: King's College.

Rumbold, G. (2003) *Ethics in nursing practice*, London: Balliere Tindall.

Secretary of State for Health (2000) *The NHS Plan: A plan for investment, a plan for reform*, Cm 4818-1, Norwich: The Stationery Office.

Secretary of State for Health (2006) *Our health, our care, our say: A new direction for community services*, Cm 6737, Norwich: The Stationery Office.

Shepherd, S. (2005) 'Social care: share issues', *Health Service Journal*, vol 115, no 5963, 7 July, pp 32-3.

Singleton, J. and McLaren, S. (1995) *Ethical foundations of health care responsibilities in decision making*, London: Mosby.

Strachan, J. (2006) 'It's time for partnerships to face the same scrutiny as everyone else', *Health Service Journal*, vol 116, no 5987, p 17.

Taylor, D. and Balloch, S. (2005) 'The politics of evaluation: an overview', in D. Taylor and S. Balloch (eds) *The politics of evaluation*, Bristol: The Policy Press, pp 1–17.

Turner, M. and Balloch, S. (2001) 'Partnership between service users and statutory social services', in S. Balloch and M. Taylor (eds) *Partnership working: Policy and practice*, Bristol: The Policy Press, pp 165–79.

# EIGHT

# Service users and ethics

*Martin Stevens and Jill Manthorpe*

## Summary

The ethical case for involving service users in service planning and delivery, and in research and evaluation, has been made on several grounds. One important set of reasons is that such involvement is ethical, as well as effective. In this chapter the ethical case for service user involvement is reviewed as well as how this involvement operates at various levels. Whether a consumerist or a more democratic or empowering approach is taken as the framework for such involvement, there are increasing principle-based justifications for user involvement.

## Introduction

Developments in health and social care in the UK, outlined in *The NHS Plan* (DH, 2000) and *Independence, wellbeing and choice* (DH, 2005), should be devised in partnership with or led by citizens with experiences of the services provided (Beresford and Evans, 1999; Peck et al, 2002). Arguments are based both on a challenge to positivist approaches underpinning the development of services (Beresford and Evans, 1999; Beresford, 2001) and also as an ethical requirement, in terms of civil rights, overcoming oppression and respect for people with disabilities (Rutter et al, 2004). In challenging traditional, linear, positivist methods, service user groups and other commentators argue that such approaches can be disempowering and miss important aspects of service users' experiences. Overall, the argument is that people who are most directly and profoundly affected by services should have a say in and be able to contribute their unique expertise to changes in such service provision. This chapter considers the challenges and the opportunities these developments imply.

## Clarifying the domain

Before moving on to the main argument, there is a need to clarify the domain. The concern in this chapter is with the development of social care and health services in general. Broadly, two strands of work can be seen to be included in this definition: managing existing or planning new services; and research that is planned, undertaken and informs direct service development. Frequently, both these sets of activities involve groups of various kinds: 'working', 'steering', 'advisory' or 'reference', to name but four varieties.

Many other forces are at play. Very often, managers and politicians also directly influence the spending on and direction of research, as well as services. Funding from charities forms a relatively small but important element of financial support for research and the voluntary sector also plays an increasing role in service provision. In parallel, other organisations, particularly commercial ones such as the pharmaceutical industry, lobby for particular research or fund their own powerful research studies and units. In many parts of social care, the commercial sector is now the dominant provider (for example, care homes for older people) and this sector's influence is now considerable if barely understood. To a variable but growing extent, service users are 'involved' in all these spheres, through being consulted, acting as consumers or purchasers of health and social care, being members of various groups or commenting through organisations run by and for service users, as well as initiating and leading projects and joining the workforce.

Consequently, complex sets of relationships develop wherein ethical issues arise, both in terms of how much influence or control service users have and also in managing the range of processes of involvement in ways that are not disempowering. These relationships will be discussed in more detail below.

The present publication has started with a discussion of general ethical issues and principles, which are central to codes of ethics in health and social care (Butler, 2002). Such concerns provide a common basis from which to discuss the ethical issues underlying the involvement of service users at all levels in service delivery, development and research. Some of the ethical dilemmas are explored that may emerge when researchers or practitioners undertake development activities and research in collaboration with service users. The chapter finishes with some practical approaches to overcome some of the ethical issues identified, arising from the authors' own experiences in many years of work in social care and health services and research and also from the literature.

## Ethics and ethical principles

Ethics can be thought of as the study of good conduct and of the grounds for making judgements about what is good conduct (Trusted, 1987; Birch et al, 2002). Approaches to ethics are commonly identified in one of two broad perspectives (Betros, 1994). First, a deontological view is one in which ethical values have a separate existence and from which rules can be derived that people ought to choose to follow, whatever the consequences. Second, there is a utilitarian perspective, in which actions are judged on the basis of their consequences for the general good. These approaches underpin sets of principles to be followed or rights to be upheld, either because of an appeal to abstract values, good in themselves, or because of their overall benefits to the greatest number. However, as Birch et al (2002) argue, such approaches reflect western and rationalistic ethics: these authors stress the reflexive and emotional aspects of ethical conduct that are important in making decisions about relationships and interactions.

Power relationships are mediated through a variety of interactions whereby ethical conduct is enacted. Consequently, identifying what is good conduct needs to take into account the variety of and bases for power relationships between individuals in any social setting. For example, in Butler's (2002) code of practice for social work research, two of the guidelines stress the need for researchers to be working in ways that em*power* others, explicitly linking ethical practice with a need to change existing power relationships.

Butler's (2002, p 243) code is based on four principles: "respect for autonomy; beneficence; non-maleficence; and justice", and a definition of scope. Butler (2002) acknowledges that this approach echoes one originally put forward by Gillon (1994) as a way of characterising health care ethics. These ethical principles of action may be applied to situations where people are mandated to intervene in the lives of others (the 'scope'), which is the common link with health care services (for examples in a particular area of practice see Manthorpe, 2001, writing of dementia care and in health care, see Vallance, 2004). Both deontological and utilitarian 'grounds' have been argued to underlie these principles, in different ways. For example, the principle of beneficence may be respected as a generally good thing in its own right (a deontological ground) or because it benefits society as a whole (a utilitarian argument).

However, other ways of characterising ethical questions call into question such formulae. These principles involve a mixture of what Trusted (1987) terms 'fundamental' and 'secondary' principles. Trusted

(1987, p 65) argues that there are two fundamental principles: "keeping trust and benevolence". Keeping trust essentially involves accepting and fulfilling obligations that are current within a particular society and covers honest and fair dealing (justice) as well as respecting the autonomy of others. Benevolence is to be "taken as the regard for the welfare of at least some others" (Trusted, 1987, p 66) and can be seen to cover Butler's (2002) principles of beneficence and non-maleficence. Although the terminology is different, with Butler's (2002) beneficence and maleficence carrying more of a stress on the impact of actions than Trusted's (1987) benevolence and malevolence, these principles are similar.

In referring to Butler's (2002) principles to illustrate ethical issues of involving service users, claims are not being made about their status as principles (see Dancy, 2004), who argues against the idea that postulating principles is a useful approach in thinking about ethics). Principles are merely being used as shorthand to identify specific ethical issues as opposed to practical matters or the interpretation of evidence which, as Trusted (1987) notes, can commonly be confused with ethical dilemmas.

The principles of autonomy (seen as a part of a general ethical obligation of keeping trust) and beneficence/non-maleficence are more clearly involved in making the general ethical case for involving service users. In the more micro-issues encountered in individual projects discussed below, the principles of justice and fair treatment emerge as important.

## Ethical case for involving service users

Involving service users can be argued to be required by three principles. First, social work, social care and health care involve balancing benefits with potential harms that Beresford (1996) argues should be a driver for service user involvement. Researchers likewise have to make difficult decisions, in terms of identifying what degree of intrusion and time commitment (that is, the potential harms of participation) can be asked of participants compared with purported benefits. This approach can be framed in terms of the principle of (or right to) self-determination or autonomy: maximising autonomy requires developments in these services to be undertaken in collaboration with people whose lives are intimately affected by any changes planned or by the evidence created by research into these areas. Gillon (1994) also connects the principles of beneficence/maleficence and autonomy or self-determination to what he calls empowerment, which is characterised in terms of the need to support service users to be more in control of their own health care.

Second, if services and research undertaken with the involvement of service users can be established as being of better quality, then such involvement is necessary in order to follow the principle of beneficence. Finally, when developing services and research, one argument is that involving service users will result in services that have the least chance of doing harm, meeting the principle of non-maleficence. However, at present there is limited evidence about the overall impact of user participation, both in terms of the ability to influence change and about whether user-influenced developments produce better outcomes (Carr, 2004). Consequently, the clearest ethical argument for involving service users rests on the principle of autonomy.

Two key ethical dilemmas presented when involving service users are worth highlighting. First, there is often a claim that the service users involved in developing services or research initiatives are not representative, which is then used as a reason to limit the level of involvement and sometimes presented as an ethical issue. If, the argument goes, such people are atypical, then a skewed perspective will be dominant and other groups will be further disempowered. Consequently, the development of services or research will be pushed in directions that favour one group over another, further disempowering those service users from groups that do not usually participate in such endeavours, thus violating the principle of non-maleficence. Furthermore this distortion would be invisible, as these projects and initiatives would be presented as having had service user involvement.

Two arguments have been used to counter this effect, both identified in the research on service user participation reviewed by Carr (2004) for the Social Care Institute for Excellence. First, professionals who take part in these endeavours do not have to be representative of professionals but are seen as having a specific role in the process. Second, people who have experienced services are likely to bring an important perspective to the table which arguably should add to the quality of plans made (see Hanley, 2005). However, such issues do present a genuine problem in involving service users, although this factor should not be used as an excuse. What has been found to be a more appropriate response is to widen the pool of both service users and practitioners involved in these processes (Carr, 2004).

Second, payment for the time service users spend working on service development can raise issues. Professionals are paid for time spent in meetings and commenting on ideas, whereas 'lay' members (including service users) are usually unpaid, which raises issues of equity and can create a barrier to participation. Removing this barrier in this way can help undermine power imbalances as an explicit value is given to the service users' contribution. There are, however, ethical issues involved in paying service users in terms of ensuring equity of opportunity (relating to the principle of justice) (see Turner and Beresford, 2005, for details of the difficulties that can then arise). It is important to ensure that a wide range of people have an opportunity to take part and that selection procedures are run fairly if payment is being offered.

## Level of involvement

Several levels of involvement have been identified (Beresford and Evans, 1999; Andrews et al, 2004). At a basic level, service users are often consulted about their views of a service or a new initiative. Usually, this approach does not involve any change in the power relationships and is very much led by providers (Andrews et al, 2004). At a higher level, service users are involved in a wide range of partnership arrangements. At its simplest, individual service users are invited to take part in appointment processes or advisory or steering groups for professionally led projects. More sophisticated and genuine partnerships between agencies and groups of service users undertake new initiatives together, in which professionals work alongside service users. At the 'highest' level of what has been termed a 'ladder' of involvement (Barnes et al, 2003; Steel, 2004) come user-controlled initiatives, including new services and research projects or programmes.

Historically, social care and health agencies have controlled decision making about the use of resources and about what and how services are delivered (Carr, 2004). Increasingly such organisations are under pressure to show the involvement of all stakeholders when bidding for funding and to meet performance indicators. However, there is still an element of discretion in terms of the level of involvement in the management of a service that is encouraged. A decision to initiate genuine partnership or to develop services on the basis of consultation only reflects different views about the appropriate relationships between service users and organisations providing services.

The level of involvement links to two types of purposes. A consumerist approach aims to improve service delivery by raising awareness of the needs and opinions of service users. Alternatively, the democratic approach aims to expand the ability of service users to make decisions about the management, running and researching of services (see Tyler, 2002, for an example of changes in maternity care).

The latter approach involves much more power sharing and empowerment and is linked to the higher levels of involvement, partnership and user-controlled initiatives.

Butler (2002, p 244) characterises the scope of operation of ethical principles as "a space in which individuals can act according to their moral conscience", focusing on moral decisions. However, Gillon (1994) also identifies a distinction in terms of the context for action. There is a difference between the personal decisions and behaviour of practitioners, which are informed by personal morality and the decisions taken at an organisational, professional or societal level; and their participation in respect of their specific roles as practitioner, manager or member of a professional group. A similar argument can be made for service users, who can operate at both an individual domain, in terms of their interactions with frontline workers and at a more abstract level, when contributing to service development or indeed influencing the evolution of ethical codes for practice and research.

As argued above, involving service users in running/planning services and research is ethically required in order fully to respect autonomy and is also viewed by service users as being essential in order to maximise benefits and minimise harms arising from care and research, thus respecting the principles of beneficence and non-maleficence. Furthermore, evidence suggests that where involvement is limited to consultation, service users report feelings of disempowerment and frustration, as their views, once consulted, are often not influential and actually are often used to 'rubber-stamp' decisions made elsewhere (Carr, 2004). Thus, limiting involvement to this level does not follow the principle of non-maleficence. Whatever the level of involvement, the key issue is to be clear about the limits, in terms both of the external pressures on agencies and also in respect of service users' choices about the extent of involvement.

## Individual interactions

Moving to a more micro-level, the ways that user involvement is structured and managed carry ethical dilemmas (Carr, 2004). In micro interactions the reflexive and emotional aspects of ethical behaviour, espoused by Birch et al (2002), have most relevance, as personal, emotional reactions can affect working partnerships. Evans, writing from her perspective as a disabled person, a commissioner of research and as a researcher, suggests how collaboration can be fruitful in evaluation (Evans and Fisher, 1999).

## Power relationships

Notwithstanding the complexities involved in all power relationships, a number of structural and practical issues tend to disempower service users in these situations. First, professional workers and researchers are often working in large organisations, which are associated with access to resources, reputation and influence. Second, service users may well associate professionals, with whom they are working in different ways, with situations in which other professionals have been very influential over their lives. Many have power to make moral and legal judgements, such as removing children or depriving a person of their liberty. People who have experienced these kinds of relationships with social work or mental health professionals may understandably experience feelings of confusion and powerlessness, when invited to work alongside the same individuals or at least their direct peers on an ostensibly equal basis.

These imbalances can be seen to work in the reverse direction in the constructions professionals may have of service users. First, service users generally are not linked to powerful organisations and thus lack the associations of power entailed (the issue of payment is also relevant here). Second, professionals often are felt to perceive the service user as someone requiring support, which carries historical connotations of powerlessness and an inability to take part in the more abstract activities involved in developing services (Carr, 2004).

Furthermore, professionals often know each other through other projects and work situations, particularly when working as a team that can create the impression of a network or pre-existing group from which non-professionals are excluded. For example, in one of the research projects with which the authors are involved, this matter was explicitly raised by several of the service users attending the advisory group meeting. The service users pointed out that the familiarity between the professionals manifested itself most clearly during the informal periods, before and after the meeting and over coffee and lunch breaks. In their view, during the more formal part of the meeting these issues were easier to manage. However, this sense of being an outsider, which can so easily and unintentionally be created, could influence the interactions throughout the whole process.

At a wider level, if an organisation has a direct role in providing social or health care, a set of issues arise related to power over the services provided to people who are involved in what could be in part a critique of the organisation.

Without transparency over the existence of these power imbalances and conscious planning to overcome the negative effects, involvement of service users may in fact be disempowering (Carr, 2004), which violates the principle of non-maleficence. Genuine involvement requires some influence and power to be shared, at least. If no efforts are made to identify and overcome these issues there is a sense in which saying that service users have been involved is misleading and the charge of tokenism can be successfully made.

Overcoming these power imbalances requires an acknowledgement of the role and expertise of service users, which raises questions about the skills and knowledge of professionals, suggesting the need to reconstruct their role. Such a reconstruction is important at the level of individual service delivery and has been developed to some degree in mental health services (for an overview see Glasby et al, 2003). The Green Paper *Independence, wellbeing and choice* (DH, 2005) stresses that service users should be placed at the centre of the process and relate differently with professionals (as has already started to a limited degree in such developments as Direct Payments or cash for care).

## Ethical involvement

Acknowledging and then raising awareness of the power imbalances and their possible consequences can possibly ameliorate their effects. Both individual support and careful planning of methods of involvement are crucial. In a review of involvement initiatives for people with dementia, Cantley et al (2005) identify the need to 'establish a baseline' at local level in order to map current activity (often not known outside agencies or beyond individual departments) to avoid duplication and confusion.

Choosing experienced service users to chair meetings is one way to overcome perceptions of power imbalance that can help create a climate in which service users' contributions are valued, in addition to a genuine alteration in power relationships. Well thought-out ground rules, explicitly enforced by those chairing meetings, can help reduce the impact of different sets of knowledge and reduce some of the problems service users face when participating in meetings. For example, asking members of meetings not to use or at least to explain all abbreviations may avoid some of the appearance of the existence of a 'secret society' with a special language, and so on. Awareness of the possibility of feelings of being excluded from the group can lead to specific measures to encourage all members to interact in the informal parts of meetings. Identifying specific people to welcome and introduce new members during these sessions could be valuable in this regard.

More sophisticated means of addressing these issues are also required. Structuring involvement methods in different ways can change the power dynamic. One approach is to consider setting up a number of sub-groups, either to have a separate service user group or to have smaller groups attended by service users and practitioners. Representatives from each group make reports to any umbrella or steering group in which all parties have an equal say in decision making.

Also of importance is that support, in the form of training or direct resources, is also given to independent groups or organisations of service users in order that these groups can take part in initiatives on a more equal footing. Training topics to be included might include basic skills such as how meetings are run or using email and more advanced training in research methods or management techniques. Not only might this approach serve to overcome some of the power imbalances described above, but would also make the best use of service users' expertise and knowledge and help broaden participation. An example is given by Maddock et al (2004), describing how a group of service users explored the effectiveness of local mental health services. These kinds of support may also facilitate user-controlled research or user-managed services, which have a very different dynamic.

## Conclusions and contemporary challenges for service users

Involvement with service delivery and research has been seen to meet ethical requirements in terms of the four principles (respect for autonomy, beneficence, non-maleficence and justice), applied across the scope of service users. Furthermore, there is an ethical case to be made in terms of involving service users in genuine partnerships and facilitating user-controlled initiatives. While we have identified ethical dilemmas involved in working in more inclusive ways, there are clear advantages and ethical imperatives.

However, in the course of the chapter, a number of challenges for involving service users in research and service development can be identified. First, as discussed above, involving service users requires funding, in terms of payments and other support. Allocating sufficient funds for service user involvement is often problematic. Second, many service user groups report 'consultation fatigue', and there is a tendency for the same service users to be involved in a large number of projects and initiatives. Third, an increased emphasis on managerialism in public services tends to ingrain power imbalances, consequently making it harder for service users to have genuine input or control in major policy developments. Managerialism also has produced an increased emphasis on professional status for groups such as social workers. While this development is not necessarily problematic, there are dangers that greater professionalism might become manifested in a greater distance between service users and professionals, making involvement more difficult to sustain.

## References

Andrews, J., Manthorpe, J. and Watson, R. (2004) 'Involving older people in intermediate care', *Journal of Advanced Nursing*, vol 46, no 3, pp 303-10.

Barnes, C., Mercer, G. and Din, I. (2003) *Research review on user involvement in promoting change and enhancing the quality of social 'care' services for disabled people*, Leeds: Centre for Disability Studies, University of Leeds.

Beresford, P. (1996) 'Challenging the "them" and the "us" of social policy research', in H. Dean (ed) *Ethics and social policy research*, Luton: University of Luton Press, pp 41-53.

Beresford, P. (2001) 'Social work and social care: the struggle for knowledge', *Education Action Research*, vol 9, no 3, pp 343-53.

Beresford, P. and Evans, C. (1999) 'Research note: research and empowerment', *British Journal of Social Work*, vol 29, pp 671-7.

Betros, S. (1994) 'Rights and the four principles', in R. Gillon (ed) *Principles of health care ethics*, New York, NY: Wiley, pp 231-41.

Birch, M., Miller, T., Mauthner, M. and Jessop, J. (2002) 'Introduction', in M. Birch, T. Miller, M. Mauthner and J. Jessop (eds) *Ethics in qualitative research*, London: Sage Publications, pp 1-13.

Butler, I. (2002) 'A code of ethics for social work and social care research', *British Journal of Social Work*, vol 32, no 2, pp 239-48.

Cantley, C., Woodhouse, J. and Smith, M. (2005) *Listen to us: Involving people with dementia in planning and developing services*, Newcastle: University of Northumbria, Dementia North.

Carr, S. (2004) *Has service user participation made a difference to social care services?*, Position Paper No 3, London: Social Care Institute for Excellence.

Dancy, J. (2004) *Ethics without principles*, Oxford: Oxford University Press.

DH (Department of Health) (2000) *The NHS Plan: A plan for investment, a plan for reform*, London: DH.

DH (2005) *Independence, wellbeing and choice*, London: DH.

Evans, C. and Fisher, M. (1999) 'Collaborative evaluation with service users', in I. Shaw and J. Lishman (eds) *Evaluation and social work practice*, London: Sage Publications, pp 101-17.

Gillon, R. (1994) 'Medical ethics: four principles plus attention to scope', *British Medical Journal*, vol 309, no 6948, pp 184-8.

Glasby, J., Lester, H., Briscoe, J., Clark, M., Rose, S. and England, L. (2003) *Cases for change: User involvement*, London: Department of Health/National Institute for Mental Health England.

Hanley, B. (2005) *Research as empowerment: Report of seminars organised by the Toronto Group*, York: Joseph Rowntree Foundation.

Maddock, J., Lineham, D. and Shears, J. with ASSERT (2004) 'Empowering mental health research: user-controlled research into the care programme approach', *Research Policy and Planning*, vol 22, no 2, pp 15-22.

Manthorpe, J. (2001) 'Ethical ideals and practice', in C. Cantley (ed) *A handbook on dementia care*, Buckingham: Open University Press, pp 186-98.

Peck, E., Gulliver, P. and Towel, D. (2002) 'Information, consultation or control: user involvement in mental health services in England at the turn of the century', *Journal of Mental Health*, vol 11, no 4, pp 441-51.

Rutter, D., Manley, C., Weaver, T., Crawford, M.J. and Fulop, N. (2004) 'Patients or partners? Case studies of user involvement in the planning and delivery of adult mental health services in London', *Social Science and Medicine*, vol 58, pp 1973-84.

Steel, R. (2004) *Involving marginalised and vulnerable people in research: A consultation document*, Involve (http://invo.org.uk/pdfs/ Involving%20Marginalised%20and%20VullGroups%20in%20 Researchver2.pdf, accessed 12/12/2005).

Trusted, J. (1987) *Moral principles and social values*, London: Routledge and Kegan Paul.

Turner, M. and Beresford, P. (2005) *Contributing on equal terms: Service user involvement and the benefits system*, London: Social Care Institute for Excellence.

Tyler, S. (2002) 'Comparing the campaigning profile of maternity user groups in Europe – can we learn anything useful?', *Health Expectations*, vol 5, no 2, pp 136-47.

Vallance, R. (2004) 'Formation in research ethics: developing a teaching approach for the social sciences', Australian Association for Research in Education Conference, University of Melbourne (www.aare.edu.au/04pap/val04020.pdf, last accessed 31/08/05).

# Section 2
## Law, management and ethics in health and social care

# NINE

# Ethical and legal perspectives on human rights

*Louise Terry*

## Summary

This chapter examines the ethical and legal repercussions of human rights legislation. The current and future potential impact on health and social care of the enshrining of the European Convention for the Protection of Human Rights and Fundamental Freedoms into British law is explored by situating the analysis within the international perspective on human rights and the work of the World Health Organisation. An ethical critique of individual rights such as the right to the highest attainable standard of health, rights to life, liberty and privacy and the right not to be subjected to degrading or inhuman treatment, among others, will be carried out by reference to existing British, European and international case law. The impact of the Freedom of Information Act is discussed.

## Rights in health and social care

Annas's (1992, p 5) argument favouring patient rights is as applicable to social care as health care: "the concept of using patient rights to make service to the individual patient the core of health care is crucial to any humane and responsive health care system". Corporate governance re-frames service delivery in the light of user rights. Service users expect information, to have their consent to care sought and their rights to confidentiality respected. The envisioning of health and social services users as active participants with an armoury of rights challenges those service providers whose ethos remains grounded on a tradition of benevolence and altruism.

Rights–based activism has been central in improving health and social care in western countries but barriers to receiving health and social care remain: health care is rationed, drugs are restricted and welfare supplicants means-tested, scrutinised and stigmatised. Individuals asserting rights (to treatment, to welfare, to die) increasingly resort to the courts. Moral rights may be re-framed as legal rights but traditional citizenship values are threatened.

Human rights legislation seeks to define parameters between the interests of the individual and the state. In health care decision making, countervailing state interests against individual autonomy include "the preservation of life, the prevention of suicide, the protection of third parties and the maintenance of the ethical integrity of the medical profession ... [because of] ... the state's power to protect the health, safety and welfare of its citizens" (Forster and Flamm, 2000, p 143). The World Health Organisation, which has a crucial role in improving health care worldwide, explains that "international human rights documents broadly fall into two categories: those which legally bind states that have ratified such conventions and those referred to as international human rights 'standards', which are considered guidelines enshrined in international declarations, resolutions or recommendations, issued mainly by international bodies" (WHO, 2005a, p 8). Since 1948, the background of international human rights has affected health and social care delivery. The WHO 2006 report will focus on working for health.

The 1948 United Nations (UN) General Assembly 30-Articled Universal Declaration of Human Rights, together with the 1966 International Covenant on Civil and Political Rights and the 1966 International Covenant on Economic, Social and Cultural Rights (ICESCR), constitute the 'International Bill of Human Rights'. Article 1 of the Universal Declaration holds that:

> All human beings are born free and equal in dignity and rights.

Article 25 states:

> Everyone has the right to a standard of living adequate for the health and well-being of himself and of his family, including food, clothing, housing and medical care and necessary social services, and the right to security in the event of unemployment, sickness, disability, widowhood, old age or other lack of livelihood in circumstances beyond his control.

The 1950 European Convention for the Protection of Human Rights and Fundamental Freedoms provides for the "collective enforcement of certain of the rights stated in the Universal Declaration", including rights to life, prohibition of torture, slavery and forced labour, rights to liberty and security, fair trial, respect for private and family life, freedom of thought, conscience and religion, to marry and prohibition of discrimination as well as the establishment of the European Court of Human Rights (ECtHR) to adjudicate claims.

Article 12 of the 1966 ICESCR recognises:

> ... the right of everyone to the enjoyment of the highest attainable standard of physical and mental health ...

and requires:

> ... the creation of conditions which would assure to all medical service and medical attention in the event of sickness.

The foundation for health tourism is evident. Governments trying to limit health and social care to genuine citizens, as costs and demand spiral, face legal challenges.

Certain groups are singled out for special protection. Article 19 of the 1989 UN Convention on the Rights of the Child (UNCRC) requires governments to take:

> ... all appropriate legislative, administrative, social and educational measures to protect the child from all forms of physical or mental violence, injury or abuse, neglect or negligent treatment, maltreatment or exploitation, including sexual abuse, while in the care of parent(s), legal guardian(s) or any other person who has care of the child.

Yet, in Britain, the 'significant harm' criteria in the 1989 and 2004 Children Acts have been interpreted in ways resulting in both the over-representation of black children in care and failures grounded in misunderstanding of different cultural mores and anti-discriminatory practice to protect vulnerable black children from harm (Brophy and Johal, 2005).

Article 24 of the UNCRC recognises:

... the right of the child to the enjoyment of the highest
attainable standard of health....

Article 10 of the ICESCR requires that:

... special protection should be accorded to mothers during
a reasonable period before and after childbirth.

Nevertheless, "local standards of care" arguments (Farmer, 2003, p 199)
justify millions of women in developing countries being without health
care during pregnancy let alone antiretroviral therapy to protect their
babies (WHO, 2005b). In China women have endured enforced
abortions (Macartney, 2005).

The Vienna Declaration from the World Conference on Human
Rights (June 1993) reaffirmed (Part II.B.6, *The rights of the disabled
person*) that:

... all human rights and fundamental freedoms are universal
and thus unreservedly include persons with disabilities.

In 1991, the General Assembly adopted 25 principles for the protection
of people with mental illness. Principle 1 holds that:

All persons have the right to the best available mental health
care, which shall be part of the health and social care system.

Principle 8 states:

Every patient shall be protected from harm, including
unjustified medication, abuse by other patients, staff or
others or other acts causing mental distress or physical
discomfort.

However, these rights are not solely premised on notions of obligations
towards the individual. Article 29 of the (1948) Universal Declaration
says:

Everyone has duties to the community in which alone the
free and full development of his personality is possible.

Arguably, we cannot "realise our potential to be good citizens or
measure up to the moral obligations that society places on us if we are

physically and mentally disabled in ways that could be corrected through proper ... care" (Butler, 1999, p 85).

## Rights: recognition and constraints

Different countries, cultures, governments and individuals "rank differently the various rights they recognise, and take different views about which emergencies or urgent social goals" justify constraints (Dworkin, 2000, p 127). Often, even in countries like Russia, "untreatable" really means "expensive to treat" (Farmer, 2003, p 214). Some people are deemed less 'worthy' than others. A North American person with Down's syndrome had to use anti-discrimination legislation to obtain a heart-lung transplant (Dingwall, 2000, p 169). In England, a decision to refuse a future kidney transplant on grounds of the patient's autism was successfully overturned (*X Hospital Trust v S* [2003] EWHC 365 [Fam]). Proving discrimination, abuse or harm by, or on behalf of, the state is most difficult for the most vulnerable. Even if someone can prove discrimination or denial of protected human rights within a courtroom, there is no certainty that the treatment or care demanded will occur. The 1998 Human Rights Act, in force from October 2000, provides that Convention rights can be enforced in British courts and tribunals. Previously, only once claimants had exhausted appeals under the domestic system could the ECtHR hear cases.

## Human Rights Act (1998)

The 1998 Human Rights Act incorporates European Convention rights (Articles 2-18, excluding Article 13) into domestic law. The ECtHR is still the court of highest appeal once domestic remedies have been exhausted. Only 'victims' (people directly affected by the act in question) can bring proceedings. If incompetent, others can act on their behalf. Since the UK ratified the Convention in 1951, many of those rights were, arguably, already reflected in law and policy. Public bodies such as NHS trusts, primary care trusts, local authorities and organisations (private or voluntary) undertaking public functions are seen as 'emanations of the state' and so subject to the 1998 Act. When making decisions concerning service users, health and social care providers have to consider whether there is any infringement of human rights and, if so, the legitimacy of doing so. The government is planning a Commission for Equality and Human Rights. The courts must interpret legislation in a way that is compatible with Convention rights.

Remedies depend on the nature of the breach and the powers of the court. Compensation may be awarded. Many wrongly expected the Human Rights Act would have a major impact on health and social care delivery in the UK. In general, the impact has been to produce piecemeal change rather than major alterations to practice.

## Article 2: The right to life

Within days of the Human Rights Act coming into force, the courts were asked to decide whether artificial nutrition and hydration could be removed from two patients in a persistent vegetative state (*NHS Trust A v M and NHS Trust B v H* [2001] Fam 348). The court held that Article 2 includes a positive obligation to give treatment if that is in the best interests of the patient but not where treatment would be futile. Since treatment withdrawal could be carried out in line with responsible medical opinion and the patients would be unaware and not suffer, Article 3 (the right not to be subjected to inhuman or degrading treatment) would not be contravened. Dianne Pretty, a motor neurone sufferer seeking protection for her husband if he assisted her suicide, failed to persuade the ECtHR that the right to life includes a right to die or that legislation prohibiting assisting suicide infringed her Article 3 rights (*Pretty v UK* [2002] 2 FLR 45).

Countries that have ratified the ECHR have a positive obligation to safeguard life. However, the right to life is, according to government ministers, subject to financial limitations; the NHS "should not have to give life-prolonging treatment to every patient who demands it because that would mean a crippling waste of resources" (Lister, 2005, p 1). The case of *Osman v United Kingdom* [2000] 29 EHRR 245 confirms that there is no positive obligation on the state to take all steps to preserve life regardless of national resources. Nonetheless, adverse publicity surrounding cases where life-saving treatments are denied can result in political U-turns regardless of the rationality of the decision or the overall impact on the degree to which government and public bodies are trusted in their decision making.

Mental health detention facilities, the police, prison services (state and private) and immigration detention/removal centres are all obliged to observe Convention rights. Lack of safe systems of work, under-trained or overworked staff may compromise standards of care. Failure to protect other patients or prisoners from fatal attacks by fellow inmates may breach Article 2. If a detainee who was known to be, or likely to be, suicidal, commits suicide, Article 2 may be involved. However, placing someone under continuous observation to prevent suicide may breach their rights to privacy under Article 8. Carers need to consider the principle of proportionality and weigh opposing rights carefully when deciding what actions to take. Unnatural deaths in custody have human rights implications and have to be investigated. Good practice means that the family should participate and investigations should be independent, open enough to allow public scrutiny and able to determine responsibility (*Jordan v UK* [2003] 37 EHRR 2).

The right to life of the unborn child was considered in the case of *Paton v United Kingdom* [1981] 3 EHRR 408. The ECtHR held that no breach of Article 2 occurred in relation to a termination involving a 10-week foetus. However, the judgment failed to clarify whether this decision was because Article 2 did not apply to the foetus or whether the right to life was not absolute because of the mother's competing human rights under Article 8 (the right to privacy).

### Article 3: The right not to be subjected to inhuman or degrading treatment

This right, which is part of the prohibition on torture, has been raised in connection with end-of-life decisions as detailed above. A minimum threshold of severity has to be reached before the Convention rights are engaged – it is not simply a matter of what the individual believes to be degrading or inhuman. In *R v A Local Authority, ex parte T* [2004] 1 FLR 601, the threshold had not been met although the case was an example of interagency working frustrating rather than safeguarding and promoting the welfare of a child.

The right not to be subjected to inhuman or degrading treatment is an absolute right and 'no qualification or excuse' is permitted: *R v (1) The Responsible Medical Officer Broadmoor Hospital, (2) The Mental Health Act Commission Second Opinion Appointed Doctor, (3) The Secretary of State for Health, ex parte John Wilkinson* [2002] 1 WLR 419 per Hale L.J. In the case of *Price v UK* [2002] 34 EHRR 1285, a severely disabled woman was detained in prison in conditions that breached Article 3. However, the context seems that if the victim is agreed by medical experts to be insensate Article 3 will not be breached (see above). This difference is distinctly unsatisfactory since, ethically, respect for people requires that even the insensate should be treated humanely and with dignity. As Hale L.J. said in *Wilkinson* (see above), "the degradation of an incapacitated person shames us all even if that person is unable to appreciate it".

The role of the social services in protecting children, older people and other vulnerable people from being subjected to inhuman or degrading treatment may raise Article 3 concerns. In *Z and Others v United Kingdom* (ECtHR, 10 May 2001), four children experienced years of parental abuse that the local authority failed to prevent. The ruling held that Article 3 (and Article 13, the right to an effective remedy, which is absent from the 1998 Human Rights Act) had been breached.

Article 3 means people lawfully deprived of liberty are still entitled to protection of fundamental human dignity. In *Keenan v UK* [2001] 33 EHRR 913, where a prisoner committed suicide, people in custody were noted to be vulnerable; further, a failure by the authorities to provide adequate medical care may breach Article 3. In considering potential breaches of Article 3 in such cases the "... vulnerability and their inability, in some cases, to complain coherently or at all about how they are being affected by any particular treatment" must be considered.

Mental health patients frequently conflict with health care professionals over treatment (Terry, 2003). The use of control and restraint by mental health workers may breach Article 3 (*McGlinchey v UK*, App No 50390/99, 29 April 2003). Likewise, the use of seclusion arguably constitutes inhuman treatment (*Munjaz v Mersey Care NHS Trust* [2003] 3 WLR 1505). The ECtHR in *Herczegfalvy v Austria* [1992] 15 EHRR 437 held that "the position of inferiority and powerlessness which is typical of patients confined in psychiatric hospitals calls for increased vigilance in reviewing whether the Convention has been complied with". Restricted ability to exercise autonomy requires greater concern for patient best interests.

In *D v United Kingdom* [1997] 24 EHRR 423, an illegal immigrant facing deportation at the end of a prison sentence successfully appealed to the ECtHR having developed terminal AIDS. If deported, D would die under "distressing circumstances". Protecting illegal immigrants' rights over genuine citizens is arguably unjust.

## Article 5: The right to liberty and security of person

The balancing of individual versus societal interests is central to mental health care. Detention of mentally disordered people frequently produces legal challenges alleging breach of Article 5. As a result of *R v Mental Health Review Tribunal, ex parte H* [2001] 3 WLR 512, the burden of proving that the criteria for detention are no longer met should not rest on the patient seeking discharge. This burden was unduly onerous given the disparity between the parties. Overstretched and underfunded community mental health provision means some discharged mental health patients have continued to be detained in hospital for several years after a ruling that these patients are suitable for conditional discharge (for example, *Johnson v UK* and *Roux v UK*, cited by DH, 2005). Mental health review tribunals, with the power to discharge patients, are often overworked, which results in delays.

## Article 6: The right to a fair and public hearing

This right affects employees facing disciplinary proceedings or professional conduct investigations and service users seeking inquiries into adverse events. The balancing of interests means not all hearings will be public. *R v Secretary of State for Health ex parte Howard* [2002] 3 WLR 738 held that private inquiries into the conduct of two doctors would not prevent further victims coming forward. In *Re G (A Child)* [2004] FLR 876, the parents were denied a fair hearing when their local authority applied for an interim care order for G rather than committing the extra funding needed to continue a residential assessment.

## Article 8: The right to respect for private and family life, home and correspondence

The right to respect for private life also includes the right to respect for personal autonomy and dignity. As held in *Pretty v UK* (see above), Article 8 covers "... the physical and psychological integrity of the person. It can sometimes embrace aspects of an individual's physical and social identity.... Article 8 also protects a right to personal development, and the right to establish relationships with other human beings and the outside world". *R v The General Medical Council, ex parte Leslie Burke* [2005] 2 WLR 431 held that dying in distress raises concerns under Article 8 as well as Article 3 since, as per *Bensaid v UK* [2001] 33 EHRR 205 (para 47), "[t]he preservation of mental stability is ... an indispensable precondition to effective enjoyment of the right to respect for private life".

In *Glass v UK* [2004] 1 FLR 1019, the ECtHR heard how David Glass, who has severe physical and mental disabilities, was given diamorphine to control pain and designated not for resuscitation by his doctors against the wishes of his mother. The doctors believed this decision was in David's best interests and that death within hours was an inevitable, although unintended, outcome. A violent confrontation occurred on the ward where hospital managers had ensured that a police officer was already present. The allegation, that David's right to life under Article 2 was breached by the doctors, was ruled inadmissible but the ECtHR held that David's Article 8 rights to respect for his private life and, in particular, physical integrity had been breached. The ECtHR criticised the managers' failure to apply to the domestic courts for a decision as to David's best interests despite obtaining a police officer in anticipation of problems. Damages were awarded to the mother for the "stress and anxiety in her dealings with doctors and officials representing the Trust as well as feelings of powerlessness and frustration in trying to defend her perception of what was in the best interests of her child".

Pregnant women have rights, under Article 8, to determine what they do with their bodies subject to conditions enshrined in national legislation, for example, in relation to abortion. This right to privacy means that the wishes of a woman who wants to terminate a pregnancy, or refuses a Caesarean section against medical advice, can prevail over the interests of the unborn child. This has the effect of denying humanness to the unborn child. Some argue that the unborn child merely has interests that crystallise into rights on birth. However, in some North American states, once a pregnancy reaches the third trimester, the interests of the unborn child may override the mother's wishes (*Norwood Hospital v Munoz* [1991] 564 2d 1017 [Mass Sup Jud Ct]).

Respect for family life has not prevented the closure of residential homes. The principle of proportionality and balancing of interests needs to be evident in all decision making. In *M v Islington London Borough Council* [2003] 2 FLR 903, the local authority, asked for accommodation and support by a woman with no residency rights, failed to consider the impact on her minor British daughter's human rights of the decision to offer plane tickets to Guyana for both individuals. The decision was quashed by the court and had to be remade.

Social services departments seeking to protect children from potential abuse may face Article 8 challenges. In *TP and KM v UK* (ECtHR, 10 May 2001), an emergency place of safety order removed a child from her mother's care, partly due to misinterpreted video surveillance evidence. The ECtHR found that Article 8 had been breached since the mother was denied the opportunity to participate in decision making following the emergency order. Removal of children soon after birth may also be held in breach of Article 8 (*P, C and S v UK* [2002] All ER 239). Balancing children's rights against parental rights is difficult particularly when social workers know that error may result in the death or serious injury of a child but hasty or ill-founded intervention may result in damaging the child–family bond, psychological harm to the child or allegations of unprofessional behaviour on the part of the social worker. The use of covert video surveillance in child protection (and potentially the protection of other vulnerable people) is hugely controversial and Department of Health guidance should be followed closely by professionals in health and social care, education and police (Terry, 2004).

## Article 9: The freedom of thought, conscience and religion

Article 9 freedoms do not mean that parental rights to adopt a particular viewpoint or religion prevail over the interests of their children. Several legal cases have involved Jehovah's Witnesses denying life-saving blood transfusions to their children, sometimes with the older child also refusing consent as in *Re E (a minor)* [1990] 9 BMLR 1. British courts will be highly unlikely to ignore medical advice that a blood transfusion is in the child's best interests. Once 18 (adult), autonomy can prevail over best interests and Article 9 and Article 8 mean that the competent patient can refuse even life-saving medical treatment as the boy in *Re E* did.

## Article 12: The right to marry and found a family

Worldwide, the reproductive rights of people with mental or learning disabilities have not, historically, been well recognised: *Buck v Bell* [1927] 274 US 200, 207, "three generations of imbeciles are enough". Greater scrutiny of sterilisation operations has developed in the UK since 1990. In *Re SL (Adult Patient) (Medical Treatment: Male Sterilisation)* [2000] 1 FLR 465, the mother of a young man with Down's syndrome failed to persuade the court that sterilisation was in his best interests.

Changes to National Health Service (NHS) provisions of in vitro fertilisation (IVF) treatment followed *R v Secretary of State for the Home Department, ex parte Miller* [2002] QB 12 and media attention. Natalie Evans, whose ex-partner withdrew consent for the use of embryos created with his sperm, has appealed to the ECtHR after failing in the domestic courts to persuade judges that the 1990 Human Fertilisation and Embryology Act consent provisions breach her rights (Parry, 2005).

Recent changes mean that civil partnerships between same-sex couples can now occur. While not strictly marriage, many of the same obligations result and so may many of the same rights such as pensions benefits. Rights to adopt children under Article 12 mean that many social services departments have removed many previous restrictions on potential adopters. The focus is becoming one of looking at the needs of the child and what potential adopter(s) can offer.

### Article 14: The prohibition of discrimination

Anti-discriminatory practice should be the foundation of health and social care. Domestic legislation is moving towards the international human rights standards seen, for instance, in the UN Principles for the Protection of Persons with Mental Illness (1991): "[t]hese principles shall be applied without discrimination of any kind such as on grounds of disability, race, colour, sex, language, religion, political or other opinion, national, ethnic or social origin, legal or social status, age, property or birth".

## Freedom of Information Act (2000, in force 2005)

This legislation provides a right of access to information held by public authorities, which should respond to written requests for all types of information within 20 working days. Reasons for requiring the information are unnecessary. Public authorities and their contractors should have a registered publication scheme where the public can easily access routinely published information. There is a duty to advise or assist people seeking information. If costs involved exceed an appropriate level the information can be refused. The legislation holds potential for greater scrutiny of the decision-making processes of government and public bodies although a number of exemptions (including relating to terrorism, health and safety or personal information) mean that not all information has to be released – a balancing act has to be carried out between the public interest in withholding information and revealing potentially sensitive information. While covered under the 1998 Data Protection Act, personal information is exempt so patient and client confidentiality will be maintained.

## Conclusions and contemporary challenges in relation to human rights

As public bodies, health and social care organisations have a duty to observe human rights, yet the need to balance individual interests, including the rights of the service provider, and consider the interests of the wider community presents dilemmas that increasingly fall to the courts to resolve. Despite international declarations and the work of the World Health Organisation and others, millions have no access to health or social care of any sort and no hope of securing their human rights. Looking to the future, as health and social care professionals develop greater ethical understanding and hone the skills needed for interprofessional care, human rights can become realities not merely aspirations.

## References

Annas, G. (1992) *The rights of patients* (2nd edn), Tolowa: Humana Press Inc.

Brophy, J. and Johal, J. (2005) 'Significant harm criteria', in Oxford Centre for Family Law Conference, 'Challenges and Opportunities faced by European Welfare States: The Changing Context for Child's Welfare', 7-8 January, Oxford.

Butler, J. (1999) *The ethics of health care rationing*, London: Cassell.

DH (Department of Health) (2005) 'Equality and human rights' (www.dh.gov.uk/PolicyAndGuidance/EqualityAndHumanRights).

Dingwall, R. (2000) 'Law, society and the new genetics', in M. Freeman and A. Lewis (eds) *Law and medicine: Current legal issues*, vol 3, Oxford: Oxford University Press, pp 159-76.

Dworkin, R. (2000) *Sovereign virtue*, London: Harvard University Press.

Farmer, P. (2003) *Pathologies of power: Health, human rights and the new war on the poor*, Berkeley, CA: University of California Press.

Forster, H. and Flamm, A. (2000) 'Legal limits: when does autonomy prevail?', in M. Freeman and A. Lewis (eds) *Law and medicine: Current legal issues*, vol 3, Oxford: Oxford University Press, pp 141-57.

Lister, S. (2005) 'Minister puts a price on the right to life', *The Times*, 19 May, p 1.

Macartney, J. (2005) 'Officials are sacked for forcing mothers to have late abortions', *The Times*, 21 September, p 41.

Parry, R. (2005) 'Woman takes frozen embryo case to European Court', *The Times*, 27 September.

Terry, L. (2003) 'The nurse's role and the NMC code of professional practice in the use of section 58 powers', *Mental Health Practice*, vol 7, no 3, pp 22-5.

Terry, L. (2004) 'The nurse's role in safeguarding children in whom illness is fabricated or induced', *Paediatric Nursing*, vol 16, no 1, pp 14-18.

WHO (World Health Organisation) (2005a) *WHO resource book on mental health, human rights and legislation*, Geneva: WHO.

WHO (2005b) *Make every mother and child count*, Geneva: WHO.

## List of statutes and Conventions

Children Act 1989, London: The Stationery Office (www.opsi.gov.uk/acts/acts1989/Ukpga_19890041_en_1.htm)

Children Act 2004, London: The Stationery Office (www.opsi.gov.uk/acts/acts2004/20040031.htm)

Data Protection Act 1998, London: The Stationery Office (www.opsi.gov.uk/acts/acts1998/19980029.htm)

European Convention for the Protection of Human Rights and Fundamental Freedoms 1950, Strasbourg, Council of Europe (http://conventions.coe.int/)

Freedom of Information Act 2000, London: The Stationery Office (www.opsi.gov.uk/acts/acts2000/20000036.htm)

Human Rights Act 1998, London: The Stationery Office (www.opsi.gov.uk/acts/acts1998/19980042.htm)

Human Fertilisation and Embryology Act 1990, London: The Stationery Office (www.opsi.gov.uk/acts/acts1990/Ukpga_19900037_en_1.htm)

International Covenant on Civil and Political Rights 1966, United Nations General Assembly Resolution 2200A (XXI), Geneva, United Nations (www.unhchr.ch/html/menu3/b/a_ccpr.htm)

International Covenant on Economic, Social and Cultural Rights 1966, United Nations General Assembly Resolution 2200A (XXI), Geneva, United Nations (www.unhchr.ch/html/menu3/b/a_cescr.htm)

United Nations Convention on the Rights of the Child 1989, United Nations General Assembly Resolution 44/25, Geneva, United Nations (www.unhchr.ch/html/menu3/b/k2crc.htm)

United Nations General Assembly Universal Declaration of Human Rights 1948, United Nations General Assembly Resolution 217A (III), Geneva, United Nations (www.un.org/Overview/rights.html)

United Nations Principles for the Protection of Persons with Mental Illness 1991, United Nations General Assembly Resolution 46/119, Geneva, United Nations (www.unhchr.ch/html/menu3/b/68.htm)

World Conference on Human Rights Vienna Declaration 1993, United Nations General Assembly A/CONF157/23, Geneva, United Nations (www.unhchr.ch/huridocda/huridoca.nsf/(Symbol)/A.CONF.157.23.En?OpenDocument)

## List of cases

*Bensaid v UK* [2001] 33 EHRR 205

*Buck v Bell* [1927] 274 US 200

*D v United Kingdom* [1997] 24 EHRR 423

*E (A Minor), Re* [1990] 9 BMLR 1

*G (A Child), Re* [2004] FLR 876

*Glass v UK* [2004] 1 FLR 1019

*Herczegfalvy v Austria* [1992] 15 EHRR 437

*Johnson v UK* (unreported) (cited in DH, 2005)

*Jordan v UK* [2003] 37 EHRR 2

*Keenan v UK* [2001] 33 EHRR 913

*M v Islington London Borough Council* [2003] 2 FLR 903

*McGlinchey v UK* App No 50390/99, 29 April 2003

*Munjaz v Mersey Care NHS Trust* [2003] 3 WLR 1505

*NHS Trust A v M and NHS Trust B v H* [2001] Fam 348

*Norwood Hospital v Munoz* [1991] 564 2d 1017 (Mass Sup Jud Ct)

*Osman v United Kingdom* [2000] 29 EHRR 245

*P, C and S v UK* [2002] All ER 239

*Paton v United Kingdom* [1981] 3 EHRR 408

*Pretty v UK* [2002] 2 FLR 45

*Price v UK* [2002] 34 EHRR 1285

*R v A Local Authority, ex parte T* [2004] 1 FLR 601

*R v The General Medical Council, ex parte Leslie Burke* [2005] 2 WLR
   431

*R v Mental Health Review Tribunal, ex parte H* [2001] 3 WLR 512

*R v Secretary of State for Health, ex parte Howard* [2002] 3 WLR 738

*R v Secretary of State for the Home Department, ex parte Miller* [2002] QB
   12

*R v (1) The Responsible Medical Officer Broadmoor Hospital, (2) The Mental
   Health Act Commission Second Opinion Appointed Doctor, (3) The Secretary
   of State for Health, ex parte John Wilkinson* [2002] 1 WLR 419

*Roux v UK* (unreported)  (cited in DH, 2005)

*SL (Adult Patient) (Medical Treatment: Male Sterilisation), Re* [2000] 1
   FLR 465

*TP and KM v UK*, 10 May 2001,  ECtHR

*X Hospital Trust v S* [2003] EWHC 365 (Fam)

*Z and Others v United Kingdom*, 10 May 2001, ECtHR

# TEN

# Multidisciplinary team practice in law and ethics: an Australian perspective

*Robert Irvine and John McPhee*

## Summary

The concept of collaborative multidisciplinary teamwork is conceived as an important catalyst and site for social and cultural transformation in the provision of health and welfare services. In increasingly diversified and pluralist health care systems, redrawing the parameters of professional practice promised opportunities for new forms of thought and action that would achieve optimal treatment outcomes and improve the experience of care for patients. Driven in part by demands for greater efficiency and effectiveness, the movement towards multidisciplinary teamwork has taken on greater urgency as an instrument by which all health care providers can be rendered more fully productive both in clinical and social terms.

In this chapter, our reflections focus on pertinent connections between legal prescriptions, ethics and teamwork in health care settings. The argument is advanced that some legal and conventional ethics discourses stand in the way of agents developing multidisciplinary collaboration and co-participation. A further contention is that multidisciplinary teamwork would benefit from more adaptive socially founded moral frameworks that emphasise the socio-relational practice of 'creating ethics'.

## Collaborative multidisciplinary teamwork

The concept of collaborative teamwork in health care settings is an indeterminate multifaceted social and moral idea. In policy and practice, teamwork covers a range of historically produced assemblages composed of different practices, ideologies and institutions. Teams can literally be 'made up' not only of health professionals but patients, their relatives and carers, self-help groups, representatives of non-governmental organisations (NGOs) and more. Team organisation ranges across interrelated occupational roles, specialities and operational methods, body systems and sites of delivery. In this chapter the term 'collaborative multidisciplinary teamwork' is used to describe a discourse that attends to the problems of professional separation, exclusion and hierarchical relations that arrest movement towards cooperation between professions, the integration of professional expertise and the coordination of professional services.

Now widely assumed in the literature is that the health division of labour involves the dominance of one group or culture by another: medical dominance has had and continues to have an enduring and significant influence on the organisation and function of health care services (Adamson et al, 1995). From the 19th century the moral and intellectual universe inhabited by the medical profession was one in which the profession claimed, in the interest of patients, exclusive moral and cognate authority to assess, adjudicate and make judgements about matters that either impacted on the profession or arose from medical techniques (Cott, 1997). This sphere of influence extended to other 'allied' professions, overseeing and coordinating most aspects of the practice of professionals working in adjacent fields

Researchers, practitioners and policy planners have advocated collaborative teamwork as an alternative logic to medical dominance; teamwork discourse remaps the parameters of professional practice, particularly medicine's traditional authority to impose order in the health division of labour (Campbell-Heider and Pollock, 1987; Gair and Hartery, 2001). Professions, subordinate to medicine, are repositioned as clinical partners in a structure of equal status exchange, adaptation and improvement so that those who are apart are brought closer together (Cott, 1997; Sculpher et al, 2002; Sicotte et al, 2002, p 993). The professional sphere is discursively represented not as an assortment of fenced-in camps, but as networks of vital, interconnected and transformative alliances. Interdisciplinary dialogue and negotiation gives shape and meaning to the idea of 'teamwork'. Immersed in a myriad of multilayered relationships, rivalries and separations dissolve as health care providers reach across occupational boundaries (see CCSC, 1996).

Developing collaborative teamwork is a far from straightforward enterprise. Perhaps it can be best represented as an accomplishment: something that is achieved only with considerable effort and skill, thought and awareness. A number of empirical studies have reported on projects and sites that have realised a certain measure of success in establishing and maintaining 'teamwork' (Patel et al, 2000; Gair and Hartery, 2001; Brown and Crawford, 2003) but which is not, however, the whole story. By and large the majority of published empirical research and anecdotal literature suggests that the discursive regimes and social practices of collaborative teamwork harbour many discontents (Campbell-Heider and Pollock, 1987; Irvine et al, 2002; Reeves and Lewin, 2004). Teams are often represented not as sites of partnership and integration but as ideologically motivated arenas of conflict (Braithwaite and Westbrook, 2005). Long after the rhetoric of collaborative teamwork was first enunciated, interactional difficulties and communication failures 'across the clinical divides' continue to be reported in the professional literature (Kroeger-Mappes, 1989; Macdonald and Smith, 2001; ABC, 2005).

## 'Captain of the ship'

Teamwork discourse brings the delimitation of jurisdiction over leadership to the fore (Sicotte et al, 2002, p 995; Braithwaite and Westbrook, 2005, p 11). Teamwork is an accomplishment whose success depends to a considerable extent on a series of highly mediated strategies for governing complex assemblages of individual conduct, collective action, technologies, space and communication. Historically, legal discourse has nurtured the idea of the doctor as the 'captain of the ship' and so defining, determining and legitimising medicine's position in professional hierarchies.

The origins of the idea are found in the historical relationship between doctor and patient. Solo practitioners dominated the health care world in the late 19th century. The compact between doctor and patient defined the health care universe. Doctors delivered care in their offices or in a patient's home, on a cash basis. Doctors were trusted and the pact was a simple one: the patient would pay in cash for the few minimal treatments that were available and the doctor would provide care even if cash was short at times. Doctors also gave charity care in hospitals. Judicially developed general, legal and ethical principles governed the relationship of a sole practitioner and patient.

As hospitals began to develop into powerful scientific institutions around the turn of the last century, the professionalisation of nursing and the advent of antiseptic surgery speeded the reorganisation of the hospital into a bureaucratic entity. In the US, the law of 'charitable immunity' was part of the indirect subsidy to protect hospitals from liability. At the same time, hospitals were relieved of tax burdens

(*McDonald v Massachusetts General Hospital* [1876] 120 Mass 432). There was also the fear that a single judgment could destroy a hospital while deterring potential patrons from seeking the health care services provided by hospitals. Essentially hospitals, as charitable institutions, had absolute immunity from any and all negligent acts of their physicians, nurses and hospital personnel. Consequently, injured patients were forced to recover from individual hospital employees who usually were unable to pay substantial damage awards. In light of this situation, courts turned to operating surgeons with hospital privileges who not only had the deepest pockets, but often the only pockets from which the injured patient could recover (Yungtum, 1995, p 379).

Even though courts had begun slowly to whittle away some of the legal protections, by the 1950s some courts created the 'captain of the ship' doctrine to reach these 'deep pockets'. The courts reasoned that physicians and surgeons were not just the best source for recovery for injured patients but, more importantly, were the only source of recovery. In *McConnell v Williams* [1949] 65 A2d 243, the Pennsylvania Supreme Court held that operating surgeons were liable for the negligent acts of all surgical personnel that occur in surgery.

In 'captain of the ship' cases, the analysis of two elements is necessary to find the physician or surgeon liable. First, the physician or surgeon must have been in charge of those assistants during the allegedly negligent act. Second, the physician or surgeon must have had control over the agent when the agent committed the negligent act. The advantage of this doctrine is the ease by which it can be applied in surgical and similar procedures, as compared to other doctrines.

Many state courts and legislatures abolished charitable immunity when hospitals began procuring comprehensive insurance coverage for their employees. With the decline in the application of the charitable immunity doctrine, these courts determined that the 'captain of the ship' doctrine was no longer necessary to compensate plaintiffs for medical malpractice. Because hospitals' 'pockets' were no longer beyond the plaintiffs' reach, many courts considered the 'captain of the ship' doctrine outdated and unnecessary.

In the UK and Australia the 'captain of the ship' doctrine (although this nomenclature was not specifically adopted) was also reflected by early court decisions. The English courts in the early 20th century emphasised the responsibility of medical practitioners and the subservient relationship of nurses and other staff. Judgments such as *Hillyer v Governors of St Bartholomews Hospital* [1909] 2 KB 820 stressed the superior responsibility of the medical profession until the 1940s when the English courts began to reassess the responsibility of hospitals and their staff. In *Cassidy v Ministry of Health* [1951] 2 KB 343, Denning L.J. commented on the earlier judgments (including *Hillyer*), and said that such judgments were motivated by a desire "to relieve the charitable hospitals from liabilities" (Kerridge et al, 2005, pp 293-4), which the hospitals could not afford.

In Australia a recent Queensland Supreme Court of Appeal case (*Langley and Warren v Glandore Pty Ltd* [1997] QCA 342) has considered the argument that a surgeon was responsible for the actions of all those in the operating theatre. The Supreme Court determined the analogy with the surgeon as the 'captain of the ship' was "not helpful". A real problem has been that surgeons liked and identified with the romantic notion that surgeons were the 'captain of the ship' and were unwilling to admit that there were activities in the operating room that were not under their control.

'Captain of the ship' has enjoyed a moment in the sun and is now dying out as courts understand that surgeons are not captains of the ship, that surgeons are never able to control everything that occurs in the operating room and that the operating team is a collaborative venture in which the members participate and contribute their expertise and talents. As Kath Melia (2001) observed in her study of Intensive Care Units (ICUs), there still may be some circumstances where time may be of the essence (such as emergency treatment or decisions within a surgical environment) where any differences of opinion must be settled quickly, without resort to outside parties, but the matter is not the case of most health care. The circumstances are not the same as the isolated 19th-century ship where there is no external authority able to resolve differences of opinion and the maritime analogy (even if still entirely applicable to the high seas) is no longer relevant in modern health care.

Yet, the case of *Langley and Warren v Glandore Pty Ltd* suggests that the 'captain of the ship' ideology continues to leave traces of the former existence in social relations and the symbolic world even after the authoritative support has been lost. Individual doctors may mobilise ideologies from another era in order to stake a claim to authority and leadership on the grounds of their legal accountability for patient care (Gair and Hartery, 2001, p 5). In such plays of discourse, the individual doctor is not stating a legal fact but making a bid for power even though such authority can only be tentatively imputed. Systematically ordered boundary marking rationales that reinforce hierarchical superiority as a valued currency are not felicitous to professional reciprocity and collaborative relationships between professions that are the hallmark of successful team functioning (RANZCP, 2002;

Brown and Crawford, 2003, p 74). Rather, brittle and not so brittle divisions are reproduced between professional groups.

## Professional ethics and teamwork

The relationship between ethics and multidisciplinary teamwork also deserves close attention. While not all aspects of teamwork are or must be ethical, this arena is morally relevant. To date, the Australian ethics literature seems to have devoted little space to discussion of collaborative teamwork. By contrast, moral conflict has emerged as a central topic in the professional literature – an interest that shows no sign of abating. The reasons for this are not hard to understand. Health care institutions are shot through with multiple subjectivities and littered with conflicting attitudes towards and beliefs about best treatment, what constitutes a 'good' outcome and how to realise the patient getting better (Gair and Hartery, 2001, pp 8-9; Macdonald and Smith, 2001). Professionals differ morally over such issues as whether foetuses count as people; the profession's role in withholding or withdrawing treatment; and telling patients the truth about their diagnosis and prognosis. Recently, Australian health care professionals have divided over the question of whether or not physicians should be authorised to prescribe the abortifacient RU-486. Organisational structures and professional cultures are not morally neutral. The research shows that individual professionals and professional groups may have fundamentally contradictory ideas about what 'teamwork' means and how teams ought to be structured (Campbell-Heider and Pollock, 1987; Cott, 1998; Sicotte et al, 2002).

Professions are well provided with a host of codes of conduct, specific occupational ethical frameworks and case studies. The discourse also does more than establish rules that articulate the individual profession's principles and methods of distinguishing between ethical and unethical ways of dealing with situations. It does more than prescribe duties that guide social actors towards expert performance of their role as well as establishing a standard by which social practices can be ordered, justified, examined and judged under peer supervision. Ethical discourses cultivate particular forms of social distinction that demarcate occupational boundaries, marking the profession off from other occupations working in the same or adjacent fields.

Our suggestion is that there are reasons to be suspicious of conventional professional ethics discourse in multidisciplinary team settings (Irvine et al, 2002). Difficulties arise when professional codes and philosophical ethics systems become sedimented into symbolically self-enclosed moral systems, for example, 'nursing ethics' 'medical ethics', 'social work ethics'. Rather than reducing social and moral distance between disciplines, these socially constructed abstractions construct a clinical world of mutually exclusive or equal but separate 'realities' that may limit the construction of positive interdisciplinary relationships.

This view is not to argue that social actors with different ethical frameworks cannot coexist in social accord. Ordinarily, health care institutions facilitate or accommodate a degree of moral pluralism. If professionals disagree about their reasons, the need for achieving rational consensus and unified action may still be seen as relevant and treated as an organising principle (Patel et al, 2000; Melia, 2001). Institutions also have ways of aligning different ethical horizons and competing social visions. Organisational culture, made up of routines, norms and forms of etiquette, regulates difference and mediates strong sub-cultural professional identity "in a way that provides for effective social cooperation without recourse to illusory 'universal answers'" (Kerridge et al, 2005, p 44).

Still, even when conflict appears to be pragmatically overcome, thus melting into collective agreement on what is right action, moral conflict over interpretation, meaning and value can not be assumed to have been resolved (Cott, 1998; Kälvemark et al, 2004, p 10). Moral disagreement is a pervasive and inevitable part of the complex social, cultural and moral terrain of contemporary health care practice and it seems pointless to pretend otherwise.

## Ethics and voice

From one ethically loaded instance to the next, debates over meaning and practice may intrude on professionals in close proximity with others who differ morally. What matters ethically is how professionals respond to others whose difference is recognised, so that actual participation in systematic interdisciplinary dialogue is extended and cultivated.

When speaking to each other, as to when, to whom and what can be said, all health care professionals face some restrictions. While subordinated groups are not completely passive, the prospects of having their voices heard are greatly diminished in situations where the practice of one profession affects other professions (Evans, 1986; Campbell-Heider and Pollock, 1987; Burke et al, 2000; Gair and Hartery, 2001, p 4; Braithwaite and Westbrook, 2005).

The goal of collaborative teamwork and thus its morality is to challenge the imposing barriers of professional power and differentiation that stifle diversity of perspectives on complex phenomena, inhibit constructive interaction or silence subaltern occupations. In situations of moral conflict, to find subordinates, including patients, adapting, making concessions or deferring to the dominant culture is not uncommon, nor is deriving their normative foundations from a medical order that delivers certainty (Adamson et al, 1995; Cott, 1997, 1998; Gair and Hartery, 2001).

## Dialogue in ethics and teamwork

Issues to do with moral disagreement and social conflict somehow need to be resolved. Macdonald and Smith (2001) argue that if collaborative multidisciplinary team practice is to be realised, then moral differences and inconsistencies must be made explicit and acknowledged. Grievances constructed in 'other minds' left to ossify, hidden behind a veil of professional prerogative, often result in breakdown and 'crises' (Skjorshammer, 2001; Braithwaite and Westbrook, 2005). There is no doubt that 'crises' can lead to remarkably bad outcomes, poor clinical performance and major service failure with disastrous consequences for patients and their families.

Certain conceptions of dialogical ethics represent an avenue for the understanding and the possible resolution of systematic difference and moral disagreement within multidisciplinary teams. While the concept of dialogue has a ubiquitous presence in social theory and philosophical ethics, the concept is much less evident in professional ethics discourse. In what must of necessity be a preliminary and schematic overview, why dialogical ethics should be taken seriously is now considered.

What is dialogical ethics and what is distinctive about this approach? Broadly speaking, dialogical ethics is a more socially informed approach to ethics that can be applied to 'ethical dilemmas' or to moral conflict. 'Dialogical ethics' is often set against other ethical perspectives so as to communicate a particular understanding of the way ethical systems and moral life is formed. According to dialogue theorists like Richard Bernstein (1998), Chris Falzone (1998) and Michael Gardiner (1996) ethics is 'dialogical' in the sense that ethical perspectives, systems of ethical belief and substantive ethical standpoints in the concrete, emerge out of actual ongoing deliberation and negotiation between 'conversational partners'. Under the scope of the dialogue perspective, ethical systems and ethical standards are localised in time, space and social power, constituted in the contact zone on the borders of professions.

The role of dialogue ethics in critical reflection and debate is to create the conditions of possibility for new ethical standpoints and languages to be forged. In this context, dialogical approaches simply displace or abandon familiar, often taken-for-granted, traditional universalistic systems of ethics, such as consequentialist and deontological systems. Rather, conventional systems are discursively repositioned and represented as background: modes of thought and practice that parties bring to their encounters with others who may disagree. These philosophical systems of the good and the right will always be subject to critical evaluation and clarification, as Bernstein (1998, p 327) describes, in dialogical ethics: "[N]o belief or thesis – no matter how fundamental … is not open to further interpretation and criticism".

There are two basic arguments for dialogical ethics: as a system of ethical belief and conduct. First of all, as a theory committed to a substantive ethical standpoint, dialogical ethics emphasises relations of mutuality, shared responsibility and answerability between disciplines in the practical world. Second, in the context of the manifold particularities of social and moral interactions that comprise teamwork, dialogical ethics provides an alternative way of thinking about ethics and dealing with ongoing problems of moral disagreement.

With regard to ethical conduct, dialogical ethics appears to construct genuine ethicality around two poles: receptivity to dialogical interactions with those who are different, 'the other' and openness to the other. Dialogical approaches emphasise movement towards greater self-disclosure and moral scrutiny in a system of exchange relations. Bernstein (1998, p 4) writes, "The basic condition of all understanding requires one to test and risk one's convictions and prejudgements in and through an encounter with what is radically 'other' and alien'. Dialogic ethics presupposes a readiness on the part of all participants, individuals and groups, no matter their position or rank, actually to articulate and justify their preferences, values, ideas, preconceptions, prejudices and actions with others who may disagree" (Bernstein, 1998, p 4; Falzone, 1998, p 60).

Thinking things through with others has particular salience in situations that are said to be characterised by the cultural, political or social domination of one group or culture by another. Power in relationships is fundamental to the field of ethics. Yet, conventional ethics has been criticised because of the failure to address the actuality of hierarchy and the operation of power (Bernstein, 1998, p 240). On the other hand, dialogical ethics appears to be more attentive to the potential for entrenched social differences to fix meanings in ways that marginalise, devalue, silence or reduce the other to a similar order. Acts of naming and representing such values as right action are not treated as the sole privilege of the few. All parties are represented as dynamic creators and producers of ethical meaning, not passive receptors of universal principles handed down from above. Through the practice of dialogue within everyday social communication, individuals and occupational groups jointly negotiate the ethical grounds of their meeting, deliberate over moral statements and establish and transform ethical standards of conduct.

Parties are oriented to the other's self-regarding considerations: they listen carefully to what the other has to say, and attempt to come to maximise their own understanding of the other's values, moral beliefs and knowledge in a common project with others (Irvine, 2005). If the parties to the encounter are unwilling to engage in critical reflection and ongoing conversation with others, then individual and collective claims to ethical responsibility, a hallmark of professionalism, are rendered suspect.

Bernstein (1998), Falzone (1998) and Árnason (2000) point out that being strongly 'other' oriented, giving alternative viewpoints the benefit of the doubt, does not rule out the possibility for moral disagreement. The mobilisation of dialogical ethics in clinical or social service setting neither requires nor guarantees a once and for all solution to every moral disagreement (Falzone, 1998, p 60). There is no "final word" (Gardiner, 1996, p 40). Moral understanding is open to continual redefinition that gives dialogue ethics a certain unfinished quality. There is, however, always the possibility that things could be different or 'otherwise'.

Stepping back from conventional, universal, foundational systems of ethics does not rule out general standards for moral conduct and secure forms of practice. "Through the dialogical encounter", Gardiner observes, "the integrity of 'difference' is always maintained, but in a manner that does not preclude the possibility of solidarity or consensus" (Gardiner, 1996, p 40). In dialogical ethics consensus represents a temporary, contingent, context-specific unity grounded on conversation.

It is not difficult to understand and theoretically accept the need for collaborative multidisciplinary teamwork. However, acceptance in principle does not automatically guarantee collaboration in practice; much needs to be done in most circumstances to develop teamwork as a way of professional life. A major challenge of contemporary health and social care is to move members of teams beyond social and symbolic boundaries posed by social and moral differentiation so that participants are better able to interact creatively and constructively with others without foreclosing different practices, stances, ways of thinking and action.

## Conclusions

Multidisciplinary teams in health and social care are complex assemblages composed of different professions, practices, values, ideologies and belief systems. Coming to terms with such complexity and multiplicity requires a sustained reflection on the interrelationship between ethics and the social collaborations, or relational forms, occurring between people in their exchanges with one another. To that end, dialogue ethics is an invention that seems especially well suited to the multifaceted social and moral conditions that make up multidisciplinary teams.

The argument in favour of dialogical ethics is advanced from two angles. First, dialogical ethics fixes the professional gaze on some of the most fundamental and vexing questions concerned with issues of power, communication and decision making in teams. Extending dialogue to ethics creates new spaces and opportunities for cognitive, perceptual and linguistically constituted differences to be aired and conflicts to be acknowledged while systematically explored. Second, underpinned by ideals of equality, co-participation and goodwill, moral deliberation and ethical decision making are cast as collective projects: something that is constantly worked on by all members of the team in dialogue. Participants may be assisted across boundaries of professional difference and hierarchy in ways that are productive to professionals and the patients and users intended to be served. This discussion should, however, be read against the background of the recognised need of substantially more focused research with professionals, patients and service users on the ethics of teamwork and moral conflict.

## References

ABC (Australian Broadcasting Corporation) (2005) 'Healthcare inquiries', *The Health Report* (www.abc.net.au/rn/talks/8.30/helthrpt/stories/s1396044.htm, accessed 11/08/2005).

Adamson, B., Kenney, D. and Wilson-Barnett, J. (1995) 'The impact of medical dominance on the workplace satisfaction of Australian and British nurses', *Journal of Advanced Nursing Care*, vol 21, pp 172-83.

Árnason, V. (2000) 'Gadamerian dialogue in the patient–professional interaction', *Medicine, Health Care and Philosophy*, vol 3, pp 17-23.

Bernstein, R. (1998) *The new constellation: The ethical–political horizons of modernity/postmodernity*, Cambridge, MA: The MIT Press.

Braithwaite, J. and Westbrook, M. (2005) 'Rethinking clinical organizational structures: an attitude survey of doctors, nurses and allied health staff in clinical directorates', *Journal of Health Service Research and Policy*, vol 10, no 1, pp 10-17.

Brown, B. and Crawford, P. (2003) 'The clinical governance of the soul: "deep management" and the self-regulating subject in integrated community mental health teams', *Social Science and Medicine*, vol 56, pp 67-81.

Burke, D., Herrman, H., Evans, M., Cockram, A. and Trauer, T. (2000) 'Educational aims and objectives for working in multidisciplinary teams', *Australasian Psychiatry*, vol 8, pp 336-9.

Campbell-Heider, N. and Pollock, D. (1987) 'Barriers to physician-nurse collegiality: an anthropological perspective', *Social Science and Medicine*, vol 25, no 5, pp 421-5.

CCSC (Central Consultants and Specialists Committee) (1996) *Towards tomorrow: The future role of the consultant*, London: BMA.

Cott, C. (1997) '"We decide, you carry it out": a social network analysis of multidisciplinary long term care teams', *Social Science and Medicine*, vol 9, pp 1411-21.

Cott, C. (1998) 'Structure and meaning in multidisciplinary teamwork', *Sociology of Health and Illness*, vol 20, no 6, pp 848-73.

Evans, M. (1986) 'Not free to be moral', *The Australian Journal of Advanced Nursing*, vol 3, no 3, pp 35-48.

Falzone, C. (1998) *Foucault and social dialogue*, London and New York, NY: Routledge.

Gair, G. and Hartery, T. (2001) 'Medical dominance in multidisciplinary teamwork: a case study of discharge decision-making in a geriatric assessment unit', *Journal of Nursing Management*, vol 9, pp 3-11.

Gardiner, M. (1996) 'Foucault, ethics and dialogue', *History of the Human Sciences*, vol 9, no 3, pp 27-46.

Irvine, R. (2005) 'Mediating telemedicine: ethics at a distance', *Internal Medicine Journal*, vol 35, no 1, pp 56-8.

Irvine, R., Kerridge, I., McPhee, J. and Freeman, S. (2002) 'Interprofessionalism and ethics: consensus or clash of cultures?', *Journal of Interprofessional Care*, vol 16, no 3, pp 199-210.

Kälvemark, S., Höglund, A., Hansson, M., Westerholm, P. and Arnetz, B. (2004) 'Living with conflicts – ethical dilemmas and moral distress in the health care system', *Social Science and Medicine*, vol 58, pp 1075-84.

Kerridge, I., Lowe, M. and McPhee, J. (2005) *Ethics and law for the health professions* (2nd edn), Sydney, Australia: Federation Press.

Kroeger-Mappes, E. (1989) 'Ethical dilemmas for nurses: physicians' orders versus patients' rights', in J. Arras and N. Rhodes (eds) *Ethical issues in modern medicine*, Mountain View, CA: Mayfield Publishing, pp 110-17.

Macdonald, G. and Smith, P. (2001) 'Collaborative working in primary care groups: a case of incommensurable paradigms?', *Critical Public Health*, vol 11, no 3, pp 253-66.

Melia, K. (2001) 'Ethical issues and the importance of consensus for the intensive care team', *Social Science and Medicine*, vol 53, pp 707-19.

Patel, V., Cytryn, K., Shortliffe, E. and Safran, C. (2000) 'The collaborative healthcare team: the role of individual and group expertise', *Teaching and Learning in Medicine*, vol 12, no 3, pp 117-32.

RANZCP (Royal Australian and New Zealand College of Psychiatrists) (2002) *Psychiatrists as team-members*, Position Statement No 47, Sydney, Australia: RANZCP.

Reeves, S. and Lewin, S. (2004) 'Interprofessional collaboration in the hospital: strategies and meanings', *Journal of Health Services Research and Policy*, vol 9, no 4, pp 218-25.

Sculpher, M., Gafni, A. and Watt, I. (2002) 'Shared treatment decision making in a collectively funded health care system: possible conflicts and some potential solutions', *Social Science and Medicine*, vol 54, pp 1369-77.

Sicotte, C., D'Amour, D. and Morecault, M.-P. (2002) 'Interdisciplinary collaboration within Quebec community health centres', *Social Science and Medicine*, vol 55, pp 991-1003.

Skjorshammer, M. (2001) 'Cooperation and conflict in hospital: interprofessional differences in perception and management of conflict', *Journal of Interprofessional Care*, vol 15, pp 7-18.

Yungtum, J. (1995) 'Case note: medical malpractice: the "captain of the ship" sets sail in Nebraska: Long v Hacker', *Creighton Law Review*, vol 29, p 379.

# ELEVEN

# Ethics and the management of health and social care

*Jeff Girling*

## Summary

Management is essentially a practical discipline that is concerned with resolving problems and making decisions about the use of resources. The common perception is that of a concern with questions of getting things done in line with the government policy of the day. However, this is only part of the story. In the increasingly complex world of health and social care, management is also concerned with questions of value and judgement. In the real world managers have to deal with conflicting demands from communities, patients/clients and a range of organisations in the local health and social care system. Contemporary management of health and social care requires a framework within which to reach decisions that are both ethically justified and practically workable. The challenge is to think ethically and to work practically.

## Introduction

Whereas ethics has attracted great interest in the context of the caring professions, it is not necessarily the first thing to come to mind whenever the management arrangements for health and social care are under discussion. On the contrary, the common perception is one of people who are at best public servants and who are at worst faceless bureaucrats who merely carry out the wishes of their political masters. A fairly typical contemporary view is that, when all is said and done, managers tend to keep their heads down and deliver what their political masters expect of them. 'Delivery' is seen as more important than independent thought and reflection.

But is it all as simple and as negative as that? This chapter suggests that perhaps it is not, and seeks to explore how and why there is plenty of scope for ethical reasoning in management contexts. In fact it does not take too much searching to find real conflicts and choices in management contexts. For example, should managers always favour cost considerations over rights? Should managers always respect confidentiality at the expense of openness? Should managers always be obedient and implement centrally driven policy even when they have strong evidence based on years of experience that it would fail? Or should they follow their conscience as doctors or social workers might do? These are real ethical dilemmas and contemporary managers are facing them in the real world.

It might even surprise some managers themselves to hear this, but the ethical issues facing them in their professional roles are actually quite complex and multitextured. Managers have to work with a whole series of perspectives held by others. These include theories such as consequentialism and duty-based ethics, notions of rights, considerations of justice, philosophies of care and concepts such as virtue (Seedhouse, 1988). These are all viewpoints that we would expect to find in the caring professions such as medicine, nursing and social work and managers need to be aware of these in order to communicate effectively with professional colleagues.

For some managers, acknowledging the existence of differing ethical perspectives can be part of what they do. They may have studied moral philosophy, or have been exposed to ethical training as part of their personal development. However, that is not the norm. Moreover it is one thing to be aware of ethical perspectives in others. It is another matter to develop a perspective to guide your own practice. It is considered here, therefore, that the search for such a framework applicable for management itself is an important and urgent development challenge.

## Three outlooks

In order to clear the way to that end, three fictional characters are introduced. They are invited to share their views on the proposition that it is desirable in principle and feasible in practice to find a way of helping managers to develop their confidence and competence in dealing with ethical matters and also in dealing with matters ethically.

Firstly, there is 'the optimist', who holds the view that in fact there has always somehow been an intrinsic ethical dimension to health and social care management. As far as the optimist is concerned there is no problem of principle. It is just a case of making more explicit that which has been tacit for so long. In fact the optimist would say that managers do not get enough credit for their integrity of purpose in making the system work within the resources available.

Secondly, there is 'the pessimist', who claims that exploring the possibility of an ethical framework is a waste of time and effort, on the grounds that ethical reasoning requires the freedom of critical thought that is simply not available to managers (Loughlin, 2002).

Thirdly, we have 'the sceptic', who thinks that the pessimist goes over the top but also that the optimist is a bit naïve. The sceptic shares with the optimist the view that in principle there is always a space for ethical reasoning. But the sceptic also feels that any ethical framework will always have to operate within well-defined parameters of policy and resource availability and that this fact will indeed constrain the scope for independent critical thinking.

The optimist wonders what all the fuss is about. After all, managers are people who must decide and act. Just as the reflective manager calls on various parts of core management theory and thinking frameworks to help improve aspects of management performance, such as business strategy or human resource management, so could having recourse to management ethics expand and make explicit their repertoire helping them to become more responsible and effective practitioners. Too often, managers are forced by deadlines and other pressures to look at a problem and simply ask, 'How can I resolve this the quickest way?'. Questions about long-term consequences, about the direct and indirect effects of the decision on others, and about whether the decision squares with their knowledge base and own sense of fairness and propriety are too often set aside. Impulsive decision making, without any apparent regard for any moral parameters, may appear decisive, but as far as the optimist is concerned, management decision making is enhanced when managers broaden their perspective beyond the immediacy of expedient resolution and look instead to principled resolution (Wall, 1989).

Just as a manager learns how to identify, weigh up and assign priorities to the financial and technical considerations that are involved in a budgetary decision, so continued exposure to ethical considerations helps the manager to identify, weigh up and assign priorities to the ethical factors that accompany the financial and technical considerations of budget setting. In that way acquiring competence in ethics is actually the development of a craft skill (Petrick and Quinn, 1997).

On listening to the optimist, the pessimist is likely to snort with contempt (or feel pity for such a self-deluding stance). Above all, the pessimist finds it incredulous for anyone to claim seriously that managers can make rational, ethical decisions congruent with the goals and objectives of the system. For that to happen it would have to be the case that the goals and objectives of the system were rational in the first place. For the pessimist this is clearly not the case. For that reason alone, irrespective of any other consideration, the management ethics project is actually doomed on philosophical grounds.

There is even more bad news, says the pessimist. When for example advice is sought on policy issues such as the distribution of scarce resources, the dice are loaded against thoroughgoing critique. Managers are expected to be practical and positive, not ethical and critical. Their contribution is to put policy into practice, to make things work, not to engage in a fundamental critique of the policy itself (Loughlin, 2002). The pessimist might say that this is nothing personal. Invoking Aristotle's distinction between 'cleverness' and 'practical wisdom', the pessimist would encourage the manager to stick to what they do best, namely deal with budgets and matters of efficiency. They are good (that is, clever) at that. However, they lack the 'practical wisdom' to look for what the goals of the health and social care system should be in the first place.

Against such negativity, the sceptic is inclined to take issue with the pessimist. It is a step too far. As far as the sceptic is concerned the pessimist could have made a much more telling impact on the discussion by simply making a case for the valuable contribution that the discipline of moral philosophy can make to the debate about the link between theory and practice. This could (and should in the future) act as a much-needed challenge to the undue expediency, opportunism and ethical inconsistency that is sometimes evident in some 'macho' management styles. But the pessimist's all-or-nothing approach is likely to reinforce the stereotype of philosophy as an ivory tower pursuit and nothing to do with the practical world inhabited by managers and other 'doers'.

Despite some of the points scored by the pessimist and bearing in mind the concerns of the sceptic, it is concluded here that all is not lost for management ethics. It is true that managerial roles are not shaped in a perfectly rational environment. The health and social care system did not suddenly appear full-blown from a rational master plan. On the contrary, it has emerged in an incremental and often turbulent manner. Yet this history does not mean that there cannot be ethical reasons for managers to behave in certain ways, and not in other ways, within such a context.

For example, needs and demands always seem to outstrip available resources. Even if it is accepted that the methodologies used to allocate these scarce resources are suboptimal this does not alter the fact that managers still have reasons to distribute resources ethically. In fact it makes the need even more pressing. Using resources efficiently (getting most output from any given set of inputs and not wasting resources) means that the resources not wasted can be allocated to other areas of need, a matter of considerable ethical relevance (Dracopoulou, 1998).

In essence, the core of the pessimist's perspective is actually a methodological claim – namely that the process of moral reasoning is a process of deduction from some set of all-embracing independent, universally valid principles. If that is the only show in town, then the management ethics project is doomed. But it is not. In fact it is possible to describe a framework that could provide the basis for helping to make the ethical dimension as to what managers do (and could do) more explicit.

## So where do we go from here?

When all is said and done, management is a practical discipline and when managers as practical people are challenged to justify any type of decision, the initial response is not necessarily to appeal to theory, but to explain the practical steps that have been taken; to assess the facts and values relevant to the case; to explore the options that have been considered or examples from past experience; the reasons given for the choice; and how to reflect on/evaluate actions and their outcomes. This is a very practical mode of practical reasoning and is perfectly applicable to use in ethical dilemmas as long as ethical principles are incorporated into the reasoning that leads up to a decision; and also that the decision maker accepts the principles in question as part of his/her practice (Thomson, 1999).

So, on that basis, managers could use something like the following approach in sorting out their responses to ethical situations (see Figure 11.1).

**Figure 11.1:** A framework for responding to ethical situations

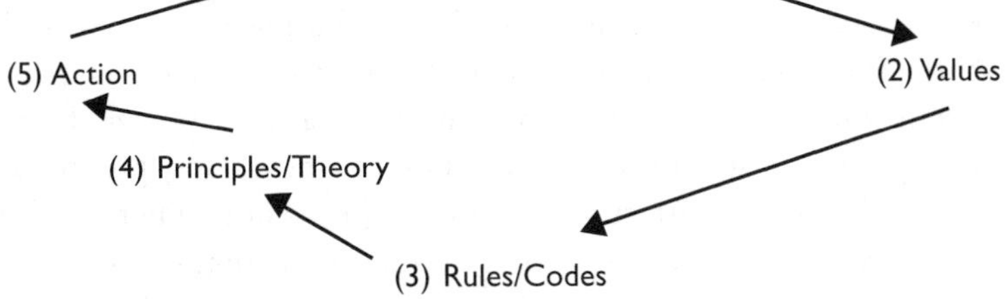

*Source:* Adapted from Newman and Brown, 1996.

1. *Intuition:* the process starts with the notion that something 'feels right' or just 'doesn't feel right'. This is the starting point because while some managers may note the existence of a possible ethics issue, they also have to assign sufficient importance to it. For example, unless it feels morally right to involve local people in decisions about commissioning services then community involvement becomes just another organisational 'must do'. Unless it feels morally wrong for there to be sexist or racist behaviours in the workplace, then the chances are that these behaviours will persist, or will not be dealt with adequately.

Exposure to, and training and practice in, interpretation can develop ethical awareness by equipping managers with the skills to interpret ethical situations adequately and accurately. However, to date, much of management education has tended to be more technically focused, with the upshot that it sometimes feels that managers are professionally socialised to prevent value conflicts from 'getting in the way' of 'business', rather than spend time sensitively resolving ethics issues as they crop up in the course of that business. It is a persisting stereotype in the health service that whereas doctors and nurses are ethical by virtue of dealing directly with patients, managers appear as either amoral or as deferential to clinical/care colleagues out of a felt sense of relative incompetence. This matter is made more difficult due to both the lack of credibility given to the now extensive body of management theory and research, together with only a weak professional requirement for managers to practise on the basis of evidence (Petrick and Quinn, 1997).

2. *Values:* it might seem slightly odd to see personal values included in the framework. However, these involve knowledge of who we are and why we value certain things on a personal level. In that sense values are closely related to the intuitive level. Values represent what it is that we truly believe, what it is we value and what kind of person and manager we want to become. Decisions based on this level make our abstract visions concrete and also connect with immediate feelings. In that way, as with intuitions, ethics can begin to feel real and felt.

3. *Rules/codes:* this stage is included in the framework with a health warning. The practical manager who wishes to deal with an ethical problem is likely to ask him/herself: are there any rules or codes that can help me? However, take note. Unlike the caring professions, management is not, strictly speaking, a profession. Therefore the definitive professional code probably does not currently exist, or if it does it certainly has no overwhelming power in the health and social

care world. Despite appearances, this relative lack is actually a positive factor as far as the framework is concerned. Most professional codes are either so general and vague that they preclude enforcement, or they are so specific that they offer little guidance in problem solving or decision making. Professional codes cannot be expected to legislate between a manager's personal values and their professional responsibilities (Davies et al, 2000). For example, a senior manager with a clinical or professional background will retain some of the instincts of their previous roles, but they cannot always rely on their previous professional codes of practice to resolve ethical dilemmas in their current management roles. Like all managers they have to reason it out for themselves, individually and collectively.

4. *Principle/theory:* moral theory only really becomes relevant when we are challenged to provide backing or more ultimate justification for underlying moral beliefs or to explain the basis for the very values or principles we use in everyday moral decision making (Seedhouse, 1998).

Authoritative sets of principles do exist that can help (Beauchamp and Childress, 1994). For example, the principle of 'beneficence' dictates that managerial actions ought to benefit those they affect. 'Non-maleficence' states that such decisions should do no harm. Respect for people instructs decision makers to preserve the autonomy of individuals and right to self-determination. The principle of justice, which has many interpretations, demands procedural fairness and an equal distribution of risks and benefits.

However, principles do not interpret themselves. Just as legal principles are developed through continuous consideration of individual cases, so do moral principles emerge gradually from reflection on particular cases. What is more, the meaning of the principles that emerge are closely tied to the factual contexts framing the issue. Principles are best seen as generalisations, as summaries of what has been decided to date within certain kinds of problem-solving situations. This is a freer process than adherence to codes and rules. Yet this also demands commitment to a process of continuous learning. It also requires explicit reflection documented as a body of knowledge for others. At present this is not sufficiently enabled or supported by a strong enough professional network in practice (Dracopoulou, 1998).

5. *Action:* the final stage in our fairly simple framework consists of working out what the impact of the decision has been or is likely to be. As well as the practical impacts, the ethical dimension requires

reflection on what has been learned about one's own decision-making processes and familiarity with ethical rules, codes, principles and theories. Hopefully the ethical manager finds him/herself in a 'learning loop' and able to discriminate between the types of decision procedures in different contexts.

In sum, such a simple framework can act as a way of illustrating a logic of management decision that is already 'out there' and which can help to make ethical thinking more directly connected to the practical world of management. While what is presented might appear as paying insufficient attention to moral theory (we can hear the pessimist sighing), in development terms it would be unproductive to urge managers to start with Grand Theory. It is much more helpful to work out from practice. However, for effective learning to take place it would require an infrastructure and practical support to enable managers to learn from each other, just as lawyers do from case law.

We now conclude this discussion by briefly reflecting on how this approach might apply in contemporary settings at the macro- and at the micro-level.

## Thinking ethically and working practically

The policy level provides a good example of an important contemporary issue. The past 20 years have seen such trends as experimentation with quasi- and actual markets in health and social care; the separation of commissioning and providing care; and an increased emphasis on regulation. This development has bred a rapid growth of top-down targets, inspection and audit regimes, bidding processes for top-down funding sources and endless streams of initiatives, plans and strategies.

Yet it does not have to be like this. Although much of organisational thinking has traditionally been influenced by top-down, command and control approaches (Seddon, 2005), it is simply not true that all managers adopt such assumptions as the more inspection and control, the better will be the outcomes. Nor is it universally accepted that top-down command structures will not have negative effects on levels of trust and staff morale. In fact, much of the recent literature would assert that an over-reliance on targets and central control are the polar opposite of what actually works in achieving client-centred practice.

Approaches that are designed on assumptions of low trust and gloomy views about human nature and values are likely to create low trust and poor motivation. They breed self-fulfilling prophecies. Yet, as the optimist would say, it does not have to be like this. People who work in public services want to focus on their purpose (clinicians want to treat patients; managers want to optimise services). Command and control may be the traditional (probably stereotypical) view of management, but in the last instance it is a normative assumption based on values that are not universal truths (Garrat, 2003).

When all is said and done, managers are faced with choice. They are undeniably accountable to higher authority. However, let us also acknowledge that they are committed to the service ethos. They feel accountable. At any particular time, they are likely to accept the legitimacy of the government of the day in its right to implement policies. At the same time, and this is the key point at the 'macro'-level, they do have choices as to how they respond to the practical challenges facing them in discharging their roles and responsibilities. In a real sense, they have a degree of moral freedom to choose how to act.

There is also plenty of scope for freedom when we turn our attention to the organisational level. Health and social care services have seen a whole host of organisational models and arrangements between and within health and social care. These include whole systems working (Attwood et al, 2003), joint planning and partnership arrangements, clinical networks as well as new types of organisations such as National Health Service (NHS)/care trusts, primary care trusts, foundation trusts and independent sector models and cooperative companies limited by guarantee operating within the public sector. Of course there are guidelines and other parameters (such as management cost limits) that are always going to be influential and that will place some constraints on what is possible. At the same time, there is still much to play for in terms of how these organisations 'come to life'.

For example, structures can be more or less centralised or decentralised. The introduction of primary care trusts in the NHS was welcomed by some and feared by others, simply on the basis of their localising tendencies. For some managers they offered the chance for greater autonomy and self-determination of frontline staff and for building links with local communities. Hence, those managers who are drawn to this set of values will welcome with open arms the opportunity for bottom–up working. At the same time, there is the need for authority and accountability. This is important to allocate the organisation's resources to achieve its objectives, stressing 'rational goals' and 'internal process' dimensions with their strong pulls towards coordination and order (and equity). While some organisations feel much more comfortable with 'the devil that they know' – that is, traditional hierarchical structures – even the most committed centralist manager has had to recognise the case literature of most successful organisations adopting non-traditional decentralised models (Attwood et al, 2003).

For some managers decentralisation 'just feels right'. It is consistent with their values (for example, sensitivity to local needs, accessibility, involvement of frontline staff etc). In the logic of the suggested framework this may be the start of a possible ethical justification as to why their organisation and its partners ought to be persuaded of the need to set about an appropriate process of organisational change and development. For the decentralist manager in a centralist organisation they might currently feel like a 'square peg in a round hole'. They have to take responsibility for their own decisions about their own careers and the type of organisation to which they wish to commit their time and energies. That is their own choice. But if they are to make an ethical choice as opposed to a self-interested choice, then they might need to use something like our reflective framework.

A self-respecting organisation will aim to balance the intellectual and technical skills necessary to carry out its formal roles, with the moral, emotional and social virtues required to build a healthy organisational culture. The sceptic might view this a bit cynically on the grounds that it just smacks of a managerialist strategy aimed at increasing productivity. To this the optimist might ask 'What's the problem with that?'. We have already pointed out that organisational efficiency can be as much of an ethical imperative as it can be a technical strategy. What is more, the optimist might say, a key feature of organising people is the development process. If we see development as an ongoing process of planned and systematic activities designed to improve individual, group and organisational performance, then the identification and nurturance of potential is a never-ending enabling responsibility of self-respecting organisations. If this takes place at individual, team and organisational levels, the beneficiaries of this are not only going to be the individuals and teams inside the organisation, but also the wider network of partner organisations and, ultimately and most importantly, the actual community and clients/patients being served (Attwood et al, 2003).

## Conclusions

If we take a look at the individual level, how would we know if we were to encounter an ethical manager? From what we have said so far, the answer would be that an ethical manager would be someone who had undertaken some form of reflective journey and had reached the point where they are seeing the relevance of moral reasoning in their 'day jobs'. Perhaps using the framework or something similar.

In the specific context of being a manager in health and social care, it is likely that a sense of justice and a sense of caring are both needed in order to be concerned both about organisational performance and viability, about eliminating and avoiding waste and about meeting needs.

This ethical dimension can still go comfortably hand in glove with other managerial attributes such as hiring and firing, setting up quality assurance systems, making firm decisions and managing change. Ethical management would neither be 'soft' management nor 'macho'. It would instead consist of the ability to discriminate right from wrong as well as the ability to discriminate between efficient and inefficient. In that way the ethical manager is able to synthesise the competing pressures of being technically competent and ethically competent. In other words the ethical manager is able to think ethically and act practically.

To sum up, the main points being made throughout this chapter are that the policy trends in health and social care provide us with a stark reminder of the desirability of a search for an appropriate ethic to help guide the practice of management. At the same time, it has been argued that there are no 'off-the-shelf' solutions. Even if there were, these should be treated with extreme caution. This is because the challenge lies very squarely before management itself. It has to find its own approach and method of formalising learning in order to enable effective managerial practice. What is offered here is best seen as a 'starter for ten'. There is much work still to be done if managers are to build on the assumption that underpins the suggested framework that ethical and general managerial decision making are interdependent and need to be recognised as such and developed together.

## References

Attwood, M., Pedler, M., Pritchard, S. and Wilkinson, D. (2003) *Leading change: A guide to whole systems working*, Bristol: The Policy Press.

Beauchamp, T. and Childress, J.F. (1994) *Principles of biomedical ethics*, New York, NY: Oxford University Press.

Davies, C., Finlay, L. and Bullman, A. (2000) *Changing practice in health and social care*, London: Sage Publications.

Dracopoulou, S (1998) *Ethics and values in health care management*, London: Routledge.

Garrat, B. (ed) (2003) *Developing strategic thought*, London: Profile Books.

Loughlin, M. (2002) *Ethics, management and mythology*, Abingdon: Radcliffe Medical Press.

Newman, D. and Brown, R. (1996) *Applied ethics for program evaluation*, London: Sage Publications.

Petrick, J. and Quinn, J. (1997) *Management ethics: Integrity at work*, London: Sage Publications.

Seddon, J. (2005) *Freedom from command and control*, Buckingham: Vanguard Education Ltd.

Seedhouse, D. (1988) *Ethics: The heart of health care*, Chichester: Wiley.

Thomson, A. (1999) *Critical reasoning in ethics*, London: Routledge.

Wall, A. (1989) *Ethics and the health services manager*, London: Kings Fund.

# TWELVE

# Ethics and the social responsibility of institutions regarding resource allocation in health and social care: a US perspective

*Mary Dombeck and Tobie Hittle Olsan*

## Summary

Like people, institutions are social structures that embody history, values, purposes, power and relationships. In the US (United States), health care contexts are defined by the health care seeker's ability to pay for services through insurance payers and by payers making services available through health care providers. Some services are provided by public funds. However, there are many people who are not eligible for any of these programmes who join the ranks of the more than 43 million in the US without insurance (IOM, 2001; Skocpol and Keenan 2005). Although unemployed people are especially vulnerable to being uninsured, many live in working families (IOM, 2001). Moreover, a disproportionate number of uninsured people are in minority ethnic and racial groups, and have very limited or no access to health care (Link and Phelan, 2005; Williams, 2005). Thus institutional structural arrangements have ethical implications because they result in disparate care and services for different populations and place ethical and moral burdens on providers. In this chapter, institutional responsibility regarding resource allocation is explored and discussed. The complexities of the US health care system are examined by describing four contexts of health care delivery, their historical background and the ethical implications of justice. Second, evidence for and examples of disparate health care in different populations are described. Third, the depersonalising effect of institutions on recipients and providers is described. Fourth, recommendations are made for moral institutional responses to these challenges.

## Four health care contexts

Almost seven out of every ten people under the age of 65 in the US subscribe to employment-based health insurance purchased through their own or a family member's employment (IOM, 2001). Many who do not fall within this context receive health care through public funds or through charitable arrangements provided by not-for-profit institutions. A context refers not to a setting, but to the social relationships, rules and structural arrangements among interconnected groups within social structures. When health care contexts are defined by health care seekers' ability to pay for services and insurance companies or health care organisations (HCOs) making services available, four contexts become apparent (see Figure 12.1):

1. Services covered by employer-provided insurance.
2. Services provided by public funds.
3. Charitable services given to the uninsured who do not qualify for private or public funds.
4. Services not covered by insurance that the health care seeker would value enough to pay out of pocket.

**Figure 12.1:** Four health care contexts

Services paid by
health insurance

| Patients paying for health care services | Employer-provided health care (eg, HCOs, Group Insurance) (1) | Service provided by public funds (eg, Medicaid) (2) | Patients NOT paying for health care services |
|---|---|---|---|
| | Services paid for out of pocket (eg complementary and alternative medicine) (4) | Charitable, philanthropic, health care services (3) | |

Services NOT paid by
health insurance

There is a constant turnover of people in these contexts. These four contexts are neither stable nor enduring. For example, when people lose their jobs they often also lose their health insurance and may qualify for some public service or resort to seeking charity care. Similarly people seeking employment always consider the availability of employment arrangements that offer health insurance coverage in order to change their situation with regard to health care payment and availability.

## 1. Employer-provided insurance

Employer-provided insurance began in the first half of the 20th century when contractual arrangements were established between industrial companies and physicians or hospitals to provide health care to employees for preset fees. These arrangements proved successful for all concerned: the workers received health care, the providers were paid and the company received the benefit of having a healthy, stable and often loyal workforce. Many partnerships that followed began experimenting with the concept of prepayment for health care. The company and employees contributed to a health care fund; the employees received health care at the discounted rates by participating physicians who were paid a preset fee for their services. These partnerships became the precursors of health insurance arrangements such as health maintenance organisations (HMOs) in operation today.

In the next three decades an unprecedented expansion of new and expensive technological inventions, drugs and other products flooded the health care arena. New facilities were built to accommodate the new modern equipment, sometimes with the help of the US government. Entrepreneurial individuals, companies and organisations inspired this expansion. There was little central planning. For example, there might be several identical expensive pieces of equipment in each of several small hospitals within one small city. The rising costs of the expansion was felt and borne by all concerned: the hospitals, the companies, the employers, the insurance companies, the employees and the government. The health care budget grew from $26.9 billion in 1969 to $993.7 billion in 1993 (Bodenheimer and Grumbach, 1998; Iglehart, 1999), with little prospect that the cost could be managed.

In 1973 the HMO Act was passed whereby the US government promoted the control of the cost of health care by concentrating on prevention, to reduce duplication of services and to reduce incentives for expensive treatments and long hospitalisations. The 1973 Act also required businesses with 25+ employees to provide HMO options to employees. The 1973 Act also provided grants and loans to develop new HMOs. The early HMOs were not-for-profit organisations. However, entrepreneurs believed that investor-owned corporations, answerable to shareholders, could not only control costs but also generate profits. Thus efforts to manage health care costs and improve health care quality evolved into enterprises to achieve these goals through market-driven methods. The entrepreneurial spirit encouraged competition among insurers and promoted the formation of integrated health care systems of providers and insurers to compete with other systems for enrollees. These ventures are susceptible to market forces, changes and crises. Some ventures succeed and others lose ground. The ones more likely to succeed are the ones that emphasise services that generate more profits, neglecting useful health care entities and services that turn out to be unprofitable.

Many people enrolled in employer-provided health insurance are satisfied with their care. Some HMOs are not-for-profit but most are for-profit organisations "with two goals that are often in conflict: providing health care to the sick and generating income for the persons who assume the financial risk" (Iglehart, 1999, p 70).

## Justice issues specific to employment-based insurance

General ethical concerns related to managed care programme models, situations and organisations have been explored elsewhere (David, 1999; Spidle, 1999; Agich and Forster, 2000; Dombeck and Olsan, 2002). More specifically with regard to the justice aspects of resource allocation, the limitations of employer-provided insurance are threefold. First, people who work and are covered by insurance may receive disparate care because they are at risk from health conditions considered by the insurer to be less profitable or too expensive to cover. Second, small companies with less than 25 employees are not required to provide health care benefits and many do not do so because of the expense. Therefore many people who are employed and their families do not have insurance coverage. The Institute of Medicine (IOM, 2001, p 40) reports that "more than 80 per cent of uninsured children and adults under the age of 65 live in working families". Third, employer-provided insurance is not available to people who are not employed, namely, the young (no longer covered by family plans), the old and the poor.

## 2. Services provided by public funds

Federal and state government programmes provide health care to older people, poor people, people with disabilities, federal employees and their families and military personnel and their families. The funds for these programmes are procured from taxation. These programmes comprise at least 40% of the entire health care budget.

In 1935, following the great economic depression, the Social Security Act, a post-retirement benefit programme, was started. Citizens pay into a fund, and receive monetary benefits at the age of 65. In 1965, two amendments to the Social Security Act established the Medicare and the Medicaid programmes. The Medicare programme provides health care for people aged 65 and older. Besides age, eligibility requirements include 10 full-time equivalent work quarters or having a spouse who has met these requirements (Finkelman, 2001). Medicare also pays expenses for people who need dialysis treatments and those judged to be disabled under the 1935 Social Security Disabilities Act.

Medicaid is a health plan for low-income individuals. Federal and state governments jointly fund this programme. The recipients of this programme are parents and children, older people and people with disabilities who need long-term care and services not covered by Medicare.

Health care for military personnel and their families is another large and very costly government programme. This is because the military health service system is not only an insurer but also a direct provider of health care. There are many hospitals and other health facilities owned and managed by the military and by the Veteran's Administration medical system. Growing expenses and old facilities in need of renovation are a current concern at this time. There is a review of all such facilities to determine which should be renovated and which should be closed, to the great consternation of veterans of the military who receive services from these facilities and the personnel who serve in these facilities.

The financial burden for health care on the federal government and on some state governments is 40-50% of the entire health care budget: "Medicare is the largest single payer in the United States" (Finkelman, 2001, p 40). There has been growing concern in this century that the cost of benefits and services provided by social security, Medicare and Medicaid are rising much faster than the amounts contributed by the present workforce into the fund. Many widely divergent solutions have been proposed for this problem that have stimulated popular and political dialogue. At one end of the spectrum are those who advocate reducing the financial burden on the federal government by cutting many Medicaid entitlements. Others advocate lowering costs by proposing that Medicaid be managed by HMOs (like employer-based insurance). President Bush proposes that people contribute to private investment accounts in addition to the publicly administered fund. At the other end of the spectrum, there are those who continue to call for the kind of total health care reform that would institute health care coverage for all citizens. The proposals and dialogue are ongoing.

### Justice issues specific to services provided by public funds

The structural arrangements that comprise the publicly administered health care services have multiple ethical implications, only a few of which can be explored fully at this time. More specifically, with regard to justice issues related to disparate resource allocation only four are mentioned here. First, Medicaid is funded by federal and state funds but is administered by states. There is a wide difference in eligibility requirements in different states. Some states set their eligibility standards in such a way that the very poor (people below the federal poverty level) are not eligible for care (Finkelman, 2001). Second, the administration of Medicaid by for-profit HMOs also dramatically reduces resources for the most vulnerable. Some payers intentionally create incentives for providers to deny, delay or avoid patients who do not generate revenue or are very costly (Torregrossa, 1996). Third, the different government agencies that service these programmes are large cumbersome bureaucracies that do not communicate with each other easily. For example, military and Veteran's Administration systems are monolithic. In case of illness, patients need to travel to appropriate facilities. The decision to close many military facilities creates a geographic burden on patients who have to travel, sometimes to a different city, to have their health care expenses covered. Fourth, when people lose their job they lose health insurance. These individuals incur large medical debts if they happen to become ill before they apply for public funds. Moreover, many who are in-between jobs are not covered by any plan. They join the ranks of the more than 43 million uninsured people. Many of these do not get any health care but some resort to charitable programmes.

## 3. Charitable health care services

A long-standing tradition of communitarian altruism exists for health care-related activities in the US. These efforts continue and have gained momentum in the 21st century because of the growing health care needs of the uninsured. Some HCOs are supported by donations from religious bodies and offer free care volunteered by health care providers and other altruistic people. President Bush, who has proposed that faith-based programmes be allowed to compete for government funds, lauds these efforts. Other not-for-profit organisations are secular. These are institutions that return portions of their revenue (exceeding expenses) back into organisational operations and services.

## *Justice issues specific to charitable health care services*

Not-for-profit hospitals that receive funding from state governments are required to provide some charity care for poor patients (O'Brien, 1996; Greenfield et al, 2003/04). These are important programmes because the uninsured having little access to ambulatory primary care wait until their illnesses are critical and commonly visit Emergency Departments. However, a survey of 23 hospitals revealed that hospitals are not forthcoming about their free care policy, thus "the availability of charity care or reduced fee care continues to be a well kept secret at far too many hospitals" (Greenfield et al, 2003/04, p 13). Those who need the service most may not know of its availability. Although charity care is an important source of health care services to the uninsured and some charitable organisations offer excellent care, there is little coordinated research on the availability, consistency or quality of health care services offered through charity. Thus even charitable resources are allocated inequitably.

## 4. Services paid for out of pocket

Some physicians, dissatisfied with the quality of care rendered under the constraints of the for-profit HMOs, have chosen to remove themselves from that system. These physicians, citing ethical concerns and potential damage to physician–patient relationships, have set up private practices where patients pay for services without the benefits of insurance.

Moreover, non-traditional health care providers have proliferated in the past decade. These providers offer services that have come to be known as complementary and alternative medicine (CAM). Therapies like acupuncture, herbal therapy, massage, Rolfing, qigong, healing touch (to name a few) have widely divergent techniques, theories and epistemologies. Yet many North Americans are visiting alternate practitioners more than primary care physicians (Ruggie, 2004).

Investigation on the reasons for the popularity of these therapies demonstrate that users of these therapies are disenchanted with contemporary medicine and see these therapies as a way of exercising control over their health care environment or a small part of it (Astin, 1998). The presence of CAM practitioners caused consternation among traditional health providers. More recently, a few physicians have aligned themselves with alternative practitioners to offer a combination of traditional and alternative therapies.

There is little coordinated research on the consistency and quality of CAM services. Recently the National Institutes of Health (NIH) has established a National Center for Complementary and Alternative Medicine to investigate the most utilised and the most popular alternative therapies. Ruggie (2004) maintains that not only is CAM extremely popular, but also that it is being mainstreamed. Ruggie's (2004) evidence shows that the popularity of CAM can be explained by its emphasis on the interpersonal relationships between practitioners and patients. Alternative practitioners spend more time with each patient and charge less than traditional practitioners. This is an important finding in a climate where both patients and providers have expressed dissatisfaction over the constraints on provider–patient relationships in the environment of for-profit HMOs. The most vulnerable populations who cannot afford health insurance also cannot afford alternative health care services, creating another context for disparate resource allocation.

## Health care disparities

Most social analysts of health care in the US agree that socioeconomic status accounts for much of the observed disparities in health care (Link and Phelan, 2005; Rosenbaum and Teitlebaum, 2005). However, others also show that racial and ethnic differences persist at equivalent socioeconomic levels for several disease categories (Williams, 1999, 2005; Mayberry et al, 2000). Many of these disparities are related to inconsistent access to health care, difficult and unhealthy living conditions and exposure to persistent stress. These findings are not surprising considering that for all groups health care preventive screening is lower among the uninsured and people with no usual source of care. In these populations, children are less likely to have recommended childhood immunisations (US DHHS, 2003). African American children have higher rates of hospitalisation for asthma. African Americans have 10% higher rates of cancer and 30% higher death rates from cancer compared to whites (US DHHS, 2003, p 39), and Hispanics have higher rates of cervical, oesophageal, gallbladder and stomach cancer compared to Euro-Americans (US DHHS, 2003, p 39). Williams (2005) believes that there are social and political barriers to improvement of health care in these populations. Williams (2005) also contends that most North Americans are unaware of the extent of health and social disparities and therefore lack the understanding and will to address them.

## Depersonalising effect of institutions

On 16 August 2005, *The New York Times* printed an article entitled 'In the hospital, a degrading shift from person to patient' (Carey, 2005). The article introduced the topic by telling the story of a patient who experienced the loss of her personhood. The author continues:

> Entering the medical system, whether a hospital, a nursing home or a clinic is often degrading. At the hospital, where Ms Duffy was a patient and at many others the small courtesies that help lubricate and dignify civil society are neglected precisely when they are needed most, when they are feeling cut off from others and betrayed by their own bodies. Larger trends in medicine have made it increasingly difficult to deliver such social niceties, experts say. Many hospital budgets are tight, and nurses are spread thin. (Carey, 2005, p A1)

This article from the popular media, part of a series on the current difficulties of health care institutions, comes close to describing the essential problem of depersonalisation in health care institutions. The article unfortunately reduces the problem of depersonalisation to the loss of "social niceties", and "small courtesies". These are the results, not the causes, of depersonalisation.

Henry (1973) describes depersonalisation as a consequence of being disconnected from one's social system. He says:

> If we view the idea of person from the standpoint of becoming a person, we perceive that all events that relate or bind one to the social system as personalising. It follows that everything that detaches a person from the social system can be depersonalising. (Henry, 1973, p 18)

## Contemporary challenges for recipients and providers

Many recipients in three of the four health care contexts described earlier demonstrate the vulnerability to loss of personhood. In the first health care context, even people with employer-provided insurance are vulnerable to being objectified as 'covered lives' representing market shares in for-profit HMOs (Abrahamson, 1996). Moreover, their health care is often governed by a corporate contract to which they were not a deciding party and through which they feel detached from their health care providers (Torregrossa, 1996). Many in the second health care context who rely on publicly funded health care do get health care, but often have to endure bureaucratic inflexibility and the insecurity of being considered not eligible for the health care they need. People in the third health care context who are not covered by any insurance and have to rely on charity care are completely detached from the system. They are simply not counted at all. Finally, the actions of people who pay out of pocket for health care and for CAM demonstrate that they value the relationship with the provider as the most important resource in a health care encounter.

Professionals also face depersonalisation in health care institutions. The physicians mentioned earlier are circumventing managed care rules detaching them from meaningful relationships with patients. Boutique medical practices give physicians control over their medical practice (Belluck, 2002).

Depersonalisation has also been identified as an ethical and moral dilemma for nurses working in home health care (Olsan, 2003). Like physicians, the business aspects of health care discount nurses' professional obligations and relationships with patients. A home care nurse referred to as Maria explained a dilemma she faced:

> "I have one guy who has cardiac problems, but he also has Alzheimer's. The HMO told me they would pay for me to do cardiopulmonary assessment only, nothing about the Alzheimer's.... They will pay for me to do cardiopulmonary assessment, but won't pay me to teach about his Alzheimer's disease or work with the family about making plans. It's a joke. His dementia affects his cardiac status, how can you not deal with it? He doesn't take his medication, he is angry, and he has rages. I know something is going to happen. Either this guy is going to hit his wife or he is going to

have an MI [myocardial infarction] and he's going to be in
the hospital."

Restricting Maria's visits to cardiopulmonary assessment shows the
damage done when professionals and patients are treated as goods and
services. Short-term profit maximisation (for example, denying visits)
subverts nurses' role obligations and simultaneously eclipses the illness
experience of patients.

In summary, under this section about the depersonalising effect of
institutions, the examples show that both patients and providers are
depersonalised and that ethical issues (such as justice and moral agency)
can arise when patients are affected by institutional structures. It is an
injustice when a patient's personhood is gained or lost over time
according to their health insurance plan (public, employer-based,
charity). A patient's personhood is also diminished when the burden
of disease is unfairly distributed among minorities and people who
are unemployed and uninsured.

From the perspective of professional depersonalisation, when
institutional policies conflict with patients' interests, health care
professionals may be unable to act according to their professional
conscience. Whenever more powerful institutions subvert professional
judgements a professional's personhood is at risk for being discounted.
Institutional subversion of personhood, however, is not inevitable in
institutional life. Institutional structures can be designed to respect
and support expressions of personhood.

## Social responsibility of institutions: the importance of personhood

Structural arrangements have ethical implications at the social,
institutional and individual levels (Glaser and Hamel, 1997). Our
examination of the complexities of the US health care system
demonstrates that the injustice issues related to inequities in resource
allocation are the result of social and institutional structural
arrangements. There is an understanding in social public discourse
that these problems need solutions through changes in public policy.
Elected officials and politically involved people continue to
contemplate, argue for and work towards changes that will reduce
health care costs and provide better health care for more people. It is
unlikely, however, that total health care reform instituting health care
coverage for all citizens will happen in the near future. However, it is
important to point out that moral responses to these challenges can be

made in the context of institutions by underscoring the importance of personhood.

Personhood is acquired gradually through social and institutional relations. A person is bound to a social system by explicit and implicit rules that assign rights and responsibilities to people. Thus, the social responsibility of institutions includes obligations related to the rights and responsibilities of recipients and providers of health care.

Wolgast (1992), a philosopher of professional and corporate personhood, argues that social systems and the context created not only affect the actions of people, but also what and who people become in institutions. Wolgast (1992, p 158) continues: "a responsible person exists only against a certain kind of background and in some contexts will disappear, but in the right background his moral dimensions and importance are enhanced".

The loss of personhood occurs when people and institutions are cut off from each other causing those involved to lose their influence on each other – as those people lose their 'voice' and institutions lose their 'hearing'. People can feel silenced or invisible when assuming a patient role. Similarly, this happens to providers whose roles as functionaries of institutions conflict with their responsibilities as health care providers. The loss of personhood also happens to HMO administrators when their function in institutions allows the evasion of social responsibility in favour of corporate earnings.

Wolgast's (1992) statement offers an indictment of institutional contexts for the loss of morally responsible personhood. However, the statement is also hopeful when pointing to the possibilities for moral and social change when institutions and people hold themselves and each other responsible.

Spencer et al (2000) propose ongoing efforts to involve people who have a stake in institutions like hospitals or managed care organisations (MCOs) in communication with each other. Stakeholders of health care institutions like patients, providers and administrators and community advocates each see their rights and responsibilities through their own ethical codes. Therefore Spencer et al (2000) recommend that stakeholders understand each other's ethical standards. Administrators cannot ignore providers' professional ethics and providers need to be aware of business ethics in order to understand the pressure on administrators.

## Conclusions and contemporary challenges

The US health care system is very complex. Institutional structural arrangements result in disparate care and services for different populations and place ethical burdens on providers. As a result, the ethical principle of justice is continuously challenged by inequities in health care. The evidence from the behaviour of patients and consumers of health care shows that patients value provider–patient relationships. These contemporary challenges need to be addressed through changes in public policy about health care. Meanwhile a response to these moral challenges is possible by preventing the loss of morally responsible personhood in institutions by enhancing the connection of people to their institutions so that socially responsible decisions are made.

## References

Agich, G. and Forster, H. (2000) 'Conflicts of interest and management in managed care', *Cambridge Quarterly of Healthcare Ethics*, vol 9, pp 189-204.

Astin, J. (1998) 'Why patients use alternative medicine: results of a national study', *Journal of the American Medical Association*, vol 279, pp 1548-53.

Belluck, P. (2002) 'Doctors' new practices offer deluxe service for deluxe fee', *The New York Times*, 15 January, pp A1, A18.

Bodenheimer, T. and Grumbach, K. (1998) *Understanding health policy: A clinical approach* (2nd edn), Stamford, CT: Appleton and Lange.

Carey, B. (2005) 'In the hospital, a degrading shift from person to patient', *The New York Times*, 16 August, p A1.

David, B. (1999) 'Nurses' conflicting values in competitively managed health care', *Image: Journal of Nursing Scholarship*, vol 31, p 188.

Dombeck, M. and Olsan, T. (2002) 'Ethics and managed care', *Journal of Interprofessional Care*, vol 16, no 3, pp 221-33.

Finkelman, A. (2001) *Managed care: A nursing perspective*, Upper Saddle River, NJ: Prentice Hall.

Glaser, J. and Hamel, R. (eds) (1997) *Three realms of managed care: Societal, institutional and individual*, Kansas City, KS: Sheed and Ward.

Greenfield, S., Guercia, R. and Kass, D. (2003/04) 'Access to health care for the uninsured on Long Island: a case study', *The Journal of the New York State Nurses Association*, vol 34, no 2, pp 9-14.

Henry, J. (1973) *On sham, vulnerability and other forms of self destruction*, London: Penguin Press.

Iglehart, J. (1999) 'The American health care system', *New England Journal of Medicine*, vol 340, no 1, pp 70-6.

IOM (Institute of Medicine) (2001) *Coverage matters: Insurance and health care*, Washington, DC: National Academy Press.

Link, B. and Phelan, J. (2005) 'Fundamental sources of health inequalities', in D. Mechanic, L. Rogut, D. Colby and J. Knickman (eds) *Policy changes in modern health care*, New Brunswick, NJ: Rutgers University Press.

Mayberry, R., Mili, F. and Ofili, E. (2000) 'Racial and ethnic differences in access to medical care', *Medical Care Research and Review*, vol 57, pp 108-46.

O'Brien, J. (1996) 'A hospital administrator's view', in E. Baer, C. Fagin and S. Gordon (eds) *Abandonment of the patient: The impact of profit-driven health care on the public*, New York, NY: Springer, pp 45-9.

Olsan, T. (2003) '"We can't be nurses anymore": depersonalising contexts and community health nurses responses to market-driven health care', Unpublished dissertation, University of Rochester, Rochester, NY.

Rosenbaum, S. and Teitlebaum, J. (2005) 'Addressing racial inequality in health care', in D. Mechanic, L. Rogut, D. Colby and J. Knickman (eds) *Policy changes in modern health care*, New Brunswick, NJ: Rutgers University Press.

Ruggie, M. (2004) *Marginal to mainstream: Alternative medicine in America*, New York, NY: Cambridge University Press.

Skocpol, T. and Keenan, P. (2005) 'Cross pressures: the contemporary politics of health care reform', in D. Mechanic, L. Rogut, D. Colby and J. Knickman (eds) *Policy changes in modern health care*, New Brunswick, NJ: Rutgers University Press.

Spencer, E., Mills, A., Rorty, M. and Werhane, P. (2000) *Organization ethics in health care*, New York, NY: Oxford University Press.

Spidle, J. (1999) 'The historical roots of managed care', in D. Bennahum (ed) *Managed care: Financial, legal and ethical issues*, Cleveland, OH: Cleveland Press, pp 11-20.

Torregrossa, A. (1996) 'Legal nightmares/remedies', in E. Baer, C. Fagin and S. Gordon (eds) *Abandonment of the patient: The impact of profit-driven health care on the public*, New York, NY: Springer Publishing Company, pp 77-86.

US DHHS (Department of Health and Human Services) and Agency for Healthcare Research (2003) *National healthcare disparities report*, Rockville, MD: US DHHS.

Williams, D. (1999) 'Race, socioeconomic status, and health. The added effects of racism and discrimination', *Annals of the New York Academy of Sciences*, vol 896, pp 173-88.

Williams, D. (2005) 'Patterns and causes of disparities in health', in D. Mechanic, L. Rogut, D. Colby and J. Knickman (eds) *Policy changes in modern health care*, New Brunswick, NY: Rutgers University Press.

Wolgast, E. (1992) *Ethics of an artificial person: Lost responsibility in professions and organizations*, Stanford, CA: Stanford University Press.

# THIRTEEN

# Ethics and charging for care

*Bridget Penhale*

## Summary

In recent years, following the implementation of the community care reforms of the 1990s, there has been an increased emphasis on charging for social care. This chapter aims to provide a brief overview concerning charging for the care of vulnerable adults, encompassing deliberation of some of the historical antecedents, together with an exploration of systems of rationing. This is followed by an examination of current practice in this area, together with issues and dilemmas raised by such practice. Further exploration, through research findings, is tied to an examination of the ethical principles involved, notably justice and equity, as well as beneficence in relation to equitable treatment. Recent and potential developments within social work and care management practice are examined, together with a consideration of the framework for prevention, provision, protection and empowerment of vulnerable adults.

## Introduction

One of the key social policy questions that has been examined over the past decade is the extent to which people should pay for their own care needs in later life, as opposed to the provision of publicly funded care for all those in need of such provision. This is a vital issue in the continuing debate concerning the financing of long-term care provision in later life. While Scotland has introduced free personal care for older people, England, Wales and Northern Ireland have introduced free nursing care in care homes but not free personal care, although the implementation of this system has varied across the different countries (Wittenberg et al, 2004). Charging older people for long-term care is an important contemporary issue, exemplified by the Royal Commission on Long-term Care (Sutherland, 1999).

Work commissioned by the Joseph Rowntree Foundation has been ongoing in this area since an inquiry concerning the costs of long-term care, which was held in 1996. More recent work concerning this matter relates to projections of both future demand and spending on long-term care, with suggestions that spending on long-term care in the UK would have to increase by around 315% between 2000 and 2051 in order to meet both real rises in the costs of care and demographic pressures, assuming that existing patterns of care, funding arrangements and rates of dependency remain unchanged over time (Wittenberg et al, 2004). In order to meet such needs, the amount spent on long-term care would need to increase from 1.4% of GDP in 2000 to around 1.8% in 2051; this assumes a real increase of 2.25% in GDP each year.

In addition, recent research has investigated attitudes towards inheritance in Britain, with a nationally representative sample of 2,000 people surveyed about their views (Rowlingson and McKay, 2005). This matter is linked with the increase in levels of home ownership in the country, which indicates that more individuals will both bequeath to family members and inherit assets from members of their family. From the survey undertaken, it would appear that many people are in favour of the idea of leaving a bequest when they die, with 9 out of 10 people reporting that they have some potential to bequeath assets. Sixty-four per cent of respondents indicated that they currently had property or savings that could be left as a bequest now if necessary, while an additional 27% stated that they might have either savings or property in the future that they could bequeath. Nonetheless, most of these individuals did not consider that older people should be careful with their money in later life simply in order to leave a bequest at death. Furthermore, 66% of survey respondents who indicated some potential to leave a bequest said that they would enjoy life and would not worry unduly about their ability to leave bequests.

On the other hand, just over a quarter of respondents reported that they would be careful with their money in order to leave some form of bequest at the time of their death, with some differences apparent across different groups of respondents (Rowlingson and McKay, 2005). Such research findings are linked to the issue of charging for social care, since individuals may choose to try and avoid paying for care in order to leave larger bequests to their relatives. Additionally, some people may not wish to sell their property in order to fund care provision, but would rather that property, in particular, is passed to family members. For example, a previous study on issues relating to inheritance and intergenerational financial transfers strongly suggests that many individuals want to leave their assets, principally property, to family members (Finch, 1995).

Charging individuals for a contribution towards the costs of their care provision is not a new phenomenon and in relation to long-term (specifically residential) care was enshrined in statute in the 1948 National Assistance Act. Part III of the Act related to residential care provision, in particular for older people, hence such provision being commonly referred to within social care as Part III accommodation, particularly during the 1970s and early 1980s. However, the introduction of charges for domiciliary and other care provision (such as day care), although permitted within the framework of the 1948 Act and the 1970 Chronically Sick and Disabled Persons Act, was largely discretionary and undertaken by some, but not all, local authority social services departments during the 1970s and 1980s. This situation pertained until the introduction of the community care reforms during the early 1990s and in particular following the implementation of the 1990 National Health Service (NHS) and Community Care Act in April 1993. Under the terms of this legislation, local authority social services, while providing more flexibility and choice of provision for service users, were also required to maximise their resources and ensure value for money from their service provision. Since that time, financial assessment of an individual's ability to contribute to care costs and the levying of charges for the provision of social care has become much more commonplace within councils with social services responsibilities (CSSRs). It is also accepted as a means of generating income for such authorities.

The issues involved in charging older people for long-term care have been of increasing importance in recent years. This outcome has been clearly evident, for example, in discussions generated by the earlier Royal Commission (Sutherland, 1999). Together with this development, there has been a welcome emphasis on obtaining the views of older people in general concerning this issue (Allen et al, 1992; Diba, 1996). It would appear that a significant number of people from older generations consider that they have already contributed to the cost of care provision through insurance contributions made during their working lives. It is necessary, here, to recall that this is the generation who consider that they were led to believe, at the inception of the welfare state in the postwar period, that care would be provided from 'cradle to grave'.

## Ethical dilemmas and charging for care

While much emphasis has been placed on the views of older people, little research has investigated the views of professionals working in this area and assessed how current charging policy is translated into practice. The research study discussed below focused on the perceptions of professionals and politicians in the statutory social services involved in assessing and charging older people who anticipated entering residential or nursing home care and legal professionals who advise such older clients (Bradley et al, 2000). More specifically, the study examined professionals' attitudes to those individuals who seek to distribute assets, possibly to 'avoid' or 'evade' residential and nursing home charges. The main objectives of the study were:

- to identify and examine the ethical dilemmas faced by these groups of professionals and how these are dealt with
- to assess the extent to which values held by the professionals may or may not give rise to conflicts of interest between themselves, their employers, older people and their relatives
- to explore the extent to which attitudes, policies and expressed practice may affect how charges are levied and payments met
- to consider the extent to which current statutory arrangements regarding charging are perceived as administratively just.

This research study explored attitudes, practices and local policy in respect of charging and assessing older people in relation to residential and nursing home care. A sample of social services practitioners (care managers) were surveyed and interviews held at a number of levels with staff from five different local authorities. Using a similar methodology encompassing postal survey and interviews, the views were also explored of a smaller number of legal professionals who advise older people and who were working in the same geographical area as the local authority practitioners. The key findings from the study by Bradley et al (2000) revolved around three main themes, which are summarised below.

### Perceptions of charging

- Half the care managers and two thirds of legal practitioners involved in the research thought that financing of residential care should be means tested.

- Almost three quarters of both groups considered that nursing care should be free (the study pre-dated the implementation of free nursing care in England and Wales).
- Local authority staff at all levels held reservations about the charging system because they perceived 'loopholes' and considered that better off and better informed individuals and families avoided charges by more effective planning of their estates.

## Ethical dilemmas in policy and practice

Within the arena of social care, practice situations involving vulnerable individuals often give rise to uncertainty and ambiguity concerning the best course of action to take. This may involve some conflict between professional and personal values for practitioners and, if this is left unresolved, it may give rise to ethical dilemmas. Banks (1995, p 5) provided the definition of an ethical dilemma that was used within the research context:

> ... a choice between two unwelcome alternatives, perhaps
> by careful consideration and deciding that one alternative
> is less unwelcome than the other.

From the findings of Bradley et al (2000), it was apparent that the area of financial assessment and charging for long-term care services is one in which such ethical dilemmas occur for practitioners, perhaps in particular for those designated as care managers who are involved in financial assessments in connection with service provision. It is necessary to acknowledge here that older people who are considering a move into long-term care may be among the most vulnerable group of service users that professionals are likely to work with. Therefore situations that provoke dilemmas for practice should not be entirely unexpected, given the sensitivity required by practitioners in this area of their work.

The four key ethical principles of beneficence, non-maleficence, justice/equity and autonomy were considered during the study as of particular relevance to the dilemmas identified and reported by practitioners (for further exploration of these principles, see Beauchamp and Childress, 1992; Manthorpe, 2001). Other ethical issues that were identified principally concerned confidentiality, coercion, advocacy and paternalism. These findings relating to ethical dilemmas have been reported more fully elsewhere (Penhale, 2002). Additionally, at the time of interviews some of the care manager respondents raised other issues that they perceived as dilemmas. The areas identified as generating the most problems and dilemmas were: advice giving, checking financial details, deprivation of assets, charge avoidance and financial abuse, some of which contain ethical dimensions (see Penhale, 2003, concerning specific issues in relation to financial abuse and charging for care). The key study findings of Bradley et al (2000) relating to ethical dilemmas were as follows:

- Most (80% of) care manager participants experienced ethical dilemmas, usually in responding to the diverse needs of older people they were working with while attempting to maintain their commitment to the local authority's procedural guidelines. This resulted in a perceived lack of clarity over their role in financial assessments; legal practitioners, by contrast, were able first and foremost to focus on the interests of their older clients and appeared to experience far fewer problems in practice.

- Most care managers experienced dilemmas in relation to the extent to which they should provide information and/or advice, particularly regarding protection of assets. Many felt uncomfortable checking personal financial details and reporting suspicions about charge avoidance and at times did not carry out these functions. Some said they might use their own discretion and rely on values of trust and confidentiality to make such decisions. Other care managers said they did regularly carry out their tasks according to the guidelines, but that there was a lack of support from senior staff. Care managers and legal practitioners were also concerned at possible abuse or pressures on older people from relatives. While legal practitioners felt comfortable in dealing with these matters, care managers were often unclear and uncertain about what to do in terms of best practice.

- Almost two thirds of care managers, compared with 15% of legal practitioners, found the issues surrounding financial assessment stressful. Those who experienced ethical dilemmas the majority of the time were significantly more likely to feel stressed about conducting financial assessments. In addition, financial assessment was generally not considered to be satisfying work by care managers (82%) or by many legal practitioners (46%).

- Over half the care managers (56%) did not feel adequately trained in financial assessments, and indicated that this affected their confidence in practice. This perceived deficit requires national and local attention. There also appeared to be a lack of clear guidance for some care managers. In contrast, the vast majority of legal practitioners (83%) felt they had received sufficient training and guidance in this area of work, helping them to avoid many potential dilemmas.

- While the majority of care managers did not want to do financial assessments, many did recognise that they were best placed to provide a holistic assessment of the older person and a sizeable group felt competent in dealing with this work.
- Some of the difficulties experienced by care managers seemed to relate to problems of role ambiguity and professional identity, as reported elsewhere (Bradley and Manthorpe, 2001). That these difficulties extend to the dimensions of ethics and values should perhaps not be too surprising, in particular given previous work in this area (Clark, 2000; Hugman, 2003) and the acknowledged difficulties concerning the professional identity of the social work and social care profession.

## Fairness and administrative justice

Although the number of authorities participating in the study of Bradley et al (2000) was relatively small (five authorities in total), a number of important findings were obtained concerning the areas of fairness and administrative justice:

- Policies, procedures and practices between local authorities appeared to vary. The reasons for these differences and the variations were not always explicit or clear, even to the staff who had to apply them.
- There was a general feeling of ambivalence by the practitioners involved towards the charging system. This ambivalence seemed to be largely due to perceptions of unfairness, lack of statutory powers to uncover evidence of fraud and to pursue charge avoidance, and a perceived lack of political will to do so. The ambivalence also appeared to relate to a concern about the failure of authorities to pursue charge avoidance and to treat all individuals in an equitable and just way.
- Most of the staff who participated in the study were sympathetic towards older people and viewed the majority as honest in their transactions.
- Discretion was recognised on all levels, but staff held differing views about the scope of it and the extent to which emphasis on discretion was matched by a commitment to pursuing collection of charges,

particularly where there appeared to be reluctance to pay, or suspicions of charge avoidance.

- Some authorities had attempted to promote internal consistency through systems or developing financial assessment as a distinct and separate or specialised role. The particular systems that had been developed attempted to resolve perceived problems of inconsistency.

Although making the rules tighter within such systems could lead to an increase in procedural fairness so that people are treated more equitably, this may well not solve the problem. For instance, if the rules are too tightly drawn, then arbitrary limits could be developed and this might well lead to even more unfairness. To achieve the best balance between the twin needs for some discretion and flexibility and rules or regulations in relation to such systems is very difficult, particularly when consistency is essential. Limiting discretion would seem to be an obvious solution to the dilemmas and inconsistencies that were identified. However, whatever new systems are devised for charging it would be helpful to build in greater transparency, quality control and openness. Application and further development of the principles of administrative justice would assist any such developments (Bradley, 2003).

## Managerial perspectives

Within social care, some authors draw distinctions between managers whose values are "rooted in social work" and those who are "general professional managers with values rooted in managerialism" (O'Sullivan, 1999, p 36). This difference implies that the two sets of values are in opposition and, also, that social workers might need to set themselves in opposition to managerial perspectives. In the study reported above by Bradley et al (2000), we found that this distinction was not so clear. Managers at middle levels of social services hierarchies expressed similar views to those supporting service users. Additionally, from a managerial perspective, they could see difficulties in applying a means-tested system at the individual level and as a means of maximising the departmental budget.

Senior managers, who were some years away from direct practice experience, also made comments about the problems associated with means testing, payment collection and charging for care. They were much more likely, however, to set the picture in a political context and referred more readily to the difficulties for departments in balancing budgets. This familiarity with day-to-day practice seems to reflect the nature of the social services workforce and the link between social workers and managers may well have its explanation in the traditional model of supervision applied in many social services hierarchies. In contrast to nursing and medicine, social work supervision appears well developed and both professional and managerial issues are taken up within the context of supervision. Despite the fact that we found that many respondents did not bring issues of financial assessment to supervision, nonetheless most practitioners reported that they had regular supervision. This evidently provided their managers with a picture of day-to-day practice and its associated difficulties. In debriefing sessions with managers held in order to feed back the results of our research, most managers appeared very familiar with the issues raised by frontline staff.

Both managers and practitioners, but also staff who work in finance sections, set the principle of equity as important in their discussions of paying for services. One consequence of the implementation of community care reforms within social care services is that despite some early attention in consideration of rationing of resources (Jones et al, 1978), the apparent relevance of equity has been much more evident within social care since 1993 (Challis and Henwood, 1994). In relation to community care, questions concerning equity arise over the distribution of public resources between different client groups, income groups, generations and localities. Yet few mechanisms exist to monitor the trends that emerge from the different ways that people get access to care and there is a risk that the consequences of this may prove divisive between differential groups of service users. This was one of the reasons for the development of Fair Access to Care systems (DH, 2003) and criteria by government in 2002.

The principle of equity has been taken up at national level in respect of variation in levels of charges and in the means of calculation for social care services. The government has begun to address concerns about how this might be operating, although the reported variations were more confined to domiciliary, day care and respite payments rather than the national figures concerning charges for residential and nursing home provision set by central government under the guidance produced for Charging for Care (DH, 2006). Nonetheless within the study of Bradley et al (2000), the issue of equity also arose in respect of decisions made at senior level about pursuit of non-payment or decisions about gifts or forms of estate planning. Like practitioners, managers saw certain problems with equal access but these appeared to be framed within a broader context:

- certain families/individuals had better access to advice on financial planning;
- some individuals had not expected to be in the position of having assets of value above the threshold for charging;
- individuals had suffered ill health or disability unexpectedly and had not had the opportunity to access advice or make plans.

For many managers such issues of access were tempered by their own knowledge of the financial facts of life. In addition, they referred to the problems that would arise if generous understanding was given to some individuals in respect of others receiving less or no services. In many respects managers' arguments reflected the minority report of the Royal Commission on Long-term Care (Sutherland, 1999). A section of the report argued that while payment for residential and nursing home care was unwelcome, if such care was to be free, it would represent a reverse discrimination by effectively redistributing money to the well-off.

In essence, managers in this area found the difficulties in dealing with financial assessment symptomatic of the general pressures that they continually face in modernising social care services, particularly perhaps in relation to adult social care. As Martin and Henderson (2001, p 1) argued:

> ... the emphasis is on ensuring that services are responsive to the needs of service users, integrated across traditional professional and organisational boundaries, effective in achieving the outcomes that both individual service users and society as a whole are seeking, and inclusive in identifying and meeting the needs of disadvantaged groups.

However, as Henwood (2005, p 33) astutely observed in relation to more recent developments concerning the government policy agenda:

> ... choice, flexibility and responsive public services can be achieved only to a limited extent within a model of the welfare state that is residual and concerned with rationing services for those most in need and least able to afford to meet those needs, and against the continuing demands for efficiency savings.

The effective achievement of objectives such as those proposed above is evidently an extremely difficult process. It also does not really deal with the potential conflicts between service users and between them and 'society', together with the different interpretations possible of what constitutes a disadvantaged group. Where practitioners (social worker or care manager professionals) are at the front line in meeting such constraints, managers stand at the centre of such conflicts in respect of financial assessments. However, our research study also demonstrated that most frontline practitioners understood the position of managers. Whereas some might view managers with a degree of cynicism, most of our respondents were sympathetic to the fact that managers were often in the position of making hard choices. In addition, managers appeared to accept that taking difficult decisions was often a choice between options, both of which might have negative consequences, particularly in relation to charging for care. Furthermore, managers also perceived that dealing with the ethical dilemmas posed by such situations and encountered by frontline practitioners in their everyday practice was part of both their role and responsibility within social care, as was the provision of support to frontline practitioners.

## Conclusions and contemporary challenges presented by charging for care

Practices in charging for care could be improved through the development of better information for care managers and older people. It is also apparent that more training for professionals in financial assessment is also necessary, together with additional procedural guidance that is perhaps more explicit and user-friendly. Moreover, development of more open and consistent systems would undoubtedly help care managers when completing financial assessments. Better levels of communication between professionals would also achieve a more open recognition of the challenges that the operation of a means-tested system undoubtedly produces. Improved training at qualifying level, together with more attention to matters concerning values and ethics, would assist them to deal better with the ethical dilemmas and associated difficulties in relation to both equity and rationing that appear so prevalent in this challenging area of work.

Sen, as reported by Sceats (2005), has proposed an ethical theory of human rights that attaches/fixes human rights not solely to legislation, but is rather premised on the basic ethical principle that every individual has claims to the attention and regard of other individuals. Human rights should therefore be considered as an articulation of social ethics, which is wholly independent of the law. This is not to deny the important and necessary connection between the law and human rights, but is indicative, rather, of the many situations in which human rights are used as a basis for social action within societies over and above considerations of the law (Sceats, 2005). Within situations of charging for care, it is necessary to both acknowledge and articulate the ethical principles concerned and then to consider these within a human rights framework, in order to ensure that older people are not disadvantaged or disempowered by the processes involved.

## Acknowledgements

The author would like to acknowledge the support and assistance of the following colleagues involved in the research study discussed within this chapter: Greta Bradley, Jill Manthorpe, Justin Gore, Alan Parkin and Nick Parry. The study was funded by the Nuffield Foundation and supported by the Association of Directors of Social Services (Research Committee) and the Law Society.

## References

Allen, I., Hogg, D. and Peace, S. (1992) *Elderly people: Choice, participation and satisfaction*, London: Policy Studies Institute.

Banks, S. (1995) *Ethics and Values in Social Work,* Basingstoke: Macmillan.

Beauchamp, T. and Childress, J. (1998) *Principles of biomedical ethics* (3rd edn), Oxford: Oxford University Press.

Bradley, G. (2003) 'Administrative justice and charging for long-term care', *British Journal of Social Work*, vol 33, no 5, pp 641-57.

Bradley, G. and Manthorpe, J. (2001) 'Charging with care', *Community Care*, 23-29 August, pp 26-7.

Bradley, G., Penhale, B., Manthorpe, J., Parkin, A., Parry, N. and Gore, J. (2000) *Ethical dilemmas and administrative justice: Perceptions of social and legal professionals towards charging for residential and nursing home care*, Hull: University of Hull Publications.

Challis, L. and Henwood, M. (1994) 'Equity in community care', *British Medical Journal*, vol 308, no 6942, pp 1496-9.

Clark, C. (2000) *Social work ethics: Politics, principles and practice*, Basingstoke: Macmillan.

DH (Department of Health) (2003) *Fair access to care services: Guidance on eligibility criteria for adult social care*, London, The Stationery Office.

DH (2006) *Charging for residential accommodation guide (CRAG)*, April, London: DH.

Diba, R. (1996) 'Meeting the costs of continuing care: public views and perceptions', *Findings in Social Care Research 84*, York: Joseph Rowntree Foundation.

Finch, J. (1995) 'Inheritance and financial transfer in families', in A. Walker (ed) *The new generational contract*, London: UCL Press.

Henwood, M. (2005) 'What's driving reform?', *Community Care*, 21–27 July, pp 32-3.

Hugman, R. (2003) 'Professional values and ethics in social work: reconsidering post-modernism?', *British Journal of Social Work*, vol 33, pp 1025-41.

Jones, K., Brown, J. and Bradshaw, J. (1978) *Issues in social policy*, London: Routledge and Kegan Paul.

Manthorpe, J. (2001) 'Ethical ideals and practice', in C. Cantley (ed) *A handbook of dementia care*, Buckingham: Open University Press.

Martin, V. and Henderson, E. (2001) *Managing in health and social care*, London: The Open University/Routledge.

O'Sullivan, T. (1999) *Decision making in social work*, London: Macmillan.

Penhale, B. (2002) 'Ethical dilemmas in charging for care: contrasting the views of social work and legal professionals', *Journal of Interprofessional Care*, vol 16, no 3, pp 235-47.

Penhale, B. (2003) 'Financial abuse and charging for care: the views of social work and legal professionals', *Journal of Adult Protection*, vol 5, no 2, pp 11-20.

Rowlingson, K. and McKay, S. (2005) *Attitudes to inheritance in Britain*, Bristol/York: The Policy Press/Joseph Rowntree Foundation.

Sceats, S. (2005) Report of Paul Sieghart Memorial Lecture, given by Amartya Sen, London, *BIHR Brief*, Summer, pp 12-13.

Sutherland, S. (1999) *With respect to old age: Royal Commission on Long-term Care*, London: The Stationery Office.

Wittenberg, R., Comas-Herrera, A., Pickard, L. and Hancock, R. (2004) *Future demand for long-term care in the UK: A summary of projections of long-term care finance for older people*, York: Joseph Rowntree Foundation.

# Section 3
## Ethics: From the start of life to the end

# FOURTEEN

# Ethical challenges and the new technologies of reproduction

*Brenda Almond*

## Summary

New discoveries in genetics, when combined with developments in assisted reproduction, have raised some important and highly contentious issues. How should the right to found a family be interpreted and to what extent is reproductive choice a private matter or a matter for public regulation? Should the protections associated with adoption be extended to assisted reproduction using donated gametes? Do individuals have a right to knowledge of their genetic identity or origins if available? Are children losing something valuable, perhaps indeed a basic human right, if those origins necessarily deprive them of a genetic link to their carers or of the experience of the mother–child or father–child relationship? Should legal regulation govern other choices made possible by PGD (pre-implantation genetic diagnosis) such as sex selection, choosing a sibling as a potential bone marrow donor for another, selecting for or against a disability? What are the ethical constraints in these cases? The conclusion drawn here is that deployment of the new technological options involves a responsibility that has not existed before to protect the welfare and rights of people at a vulnerable stage of existence when they are unable to protect themselves.

## Right to found a family: private choice or public issue?

Advances in reproductive medicine offer unprecedented control to individuals over their reproductive options. For those who want it, reproduction can now be separated from sex and personal relations. The new technologies have also made it possible, through the transfer of human reproductive material (embryos or gametes, eggs and sperm), for children to be born to people to whom they are not genetically related. These children may thus be cut off in an unprecedented way from the wider network of genetic relations; siblings, half-siblings, grandparents, aunts, cousins and others who previously contributed to a person's sense of identity and who made up the wider notion of family.

This raises many questions. The fundamental underlying debate, however, is about how we conceive of 'family'. On one side of this debate is the idea of the family as fundamentally a biological concept and on the other that of family as a social and legal construct. As far as the first is concerned, it is worth pointing out that 'family' in the biological sense of a couple and their offspring is common to many species and so is a natural presumption in the case of human beings. While it may be legally convenient to regard the family as a purely social concept, the science of genetics is providing growing evidence of the importance of biological factors and the complex functioning of genes. Socially, too, individuals are increasingly interested in knowing their own complex genetic background as a way of understanding their own identity.

Until now, the distinction between the biological and the social view of the family would have been of little more than theoretical interest, but, since the birth of the first test-tube baby, Louise Brown, in 1978, it has acquired more practical importance and has brought new and unfamiliar ethical dilemmas. For parenthood has become a divisible concept: it has become necessary to distinguish between genetic, social and legal fatherhood, with motherhood facing a further possible division between the mother who supplies the egg from which the child develops and the mother who gives birth to the child. Since embryos can be frozen and then stored for long periods, children can be born years after conception and even after the death of one or both of their biological parents. Nor do reproductive possibilities end here, as scientific developments open up new and equally contentious frontiers for exploration. In particular, embryos can have other uses, including supplying stem cells for some dramatic new medical possibilities.

In the UK there was an early acceptance of the need for some form of regulation of this burgeoning field. Following a report commissioned by the government and chaired by the philosopher Mary Warnock, the 1990 Human Fertilisation and Embryology Act established principles governing assisted reproduction and set up an authority, the HFEA (Human Fertilisation and Embryology Authority), to inspect and regulate clinics carrying out assisted reproduction (Warnock, 1985).

In the US, in contrast, while federally funded research in this area is subject to control, the sale of gametes, embryos and services can be freely advertised. Some believe a cautionary approach is necessary where the untested social experiments made possible by the new reproductive technologies are concerned. Others see these technologies as offering the opportunity for the family to take new forms. Dismissing the traditional nuclear family – a man and a woman raising their own biological offspring – as an outdated concept, they may see the new opportunities as based in widely recognised human rights, in particular the right to privacy, and the right to found a family. Often cited are Article 8 of the 1950 European Convention for the Protection of Human Rights and Fundamental Freedoms: "Everyone has the right to respect for his private and family life, his home and his correspondence", and Article 16 of the 1948 United Nations (UN) Declaration of Human Rights: "Men and women of full age, without any limitation due to race, nationality or religion, have the right to marry and to found a family" (UN, 1948; Council of Europe, 1950).

How should these rights be interpreted? According to some influential commentators, a right to procreative autonomy is part of our democratic presumptions, since a constitution that guarantees religious freedom protects reproductive choices based on moral grounds (Dworkin, 1993). While Ronald Dworkin advanced this argument in relation to abortion, and so was concerned with a right not to reproduce, others have taken the argument further. John Harris believes that the principle of reproductive autonomy can be taken to cover the right to reproduce in many of the novel ways made possible by the new reproductive technologies (Harris, 1998). In contrast, the American legal philosopher, John Robertson, uses the principle of reproductive choice to defend various kinds of 'collaborative reproduction' as well as commissioned pregnancies, paid adoptions and similar contracts (Robertson, 1996).

How strong is the case for extending the interpretation of reproductive choice in the way these commentators propose? Whether reproductive rights of a novel sort can give complete freedom to some to do whatever they want must depend on whether or not there are other claimants with conflicting rights to be considered. It is for this reason that the argument that moral and religious belief make this an area of complete freedom of choice cannot be sustained. The context is one in which it is intended that children will in the end be involved. Those children will have a perspective and it may need to be considered in advance.

Often the complexity of the debate is missed because separate aspects of the reasoning about reproductive choice are not distinguished. One aspect, which the international consensus about human rights certainly supports, is a defence of the freedom of two individuals (who, prior to the new technologies, must have been a male and a female) to marry and have children together. Another is the possibility of using the new technologies to bring children into the world who are not genetically related to those who will form their immediate circle. This immediately adds to the number of stakeholders or concerned individuals and changes the role and responsibilities of the decision makers, who include clinicians and other health professionals as well as the would-be parent or parents. Where donated gametes are involved, it could be claimed that the situation is in a significant way analogous to adoption, and that this justifies applying at least some of the safeguards that are usual in that case. Indeed, those who donate gametes probably do so on the assumption that fair consideration is given to the interests of the child, so they, too, may be regarded as stakeholders in the debate. This need not be, as is often suggested, to ask doctors to sit in judgement on would-be parents. It is simply to recognise that children are the most vulnerable of all human beings and that this places a special burden of responsibility on all those who play a part in shaping their future. They cannot be viewed simply as commodities medically generated to satisfy the needs or desires of adults. As another commentator has put this, a person cannot be the object of someone else's right – there cannot be a right to acquire a human being (Ryan, 1990).

## Future children, future rights?

Assisted reproduction involving donation of gametes opens the door to parenthood for many for whom it would previously have been closed. These include single parents, older women, lesbians, gay men or cooperating groups of other kinds. But the importance of genetic relations – grandparents, aunts, uncles, cousins, to say nothing of ancestors and descendants – cannot simply be written off. Not only are they important in the lives of individuals, they have also historically supplied the webbing underpinning a culture. So there is also a child's perspective, when children created in new ways are deprived of the biological network that children conceived and born in the ordinary way are able to take for granted.

In the case of children born by assisted reproduction, however, people sometimes speak as if they believe there is a queue of children waiting in limbo for a chance to be born, so that the onus is on those who stop them being born to justify their decision. They assume that where a possible human life is at issue, existence is bound to be the better option, no matter what the circumstances. But no one is injured by not being conceived, and while most people can imagine what it would be like to wish they had never been born, it is impossible to imagine regretting not having even been conceived.

So while there is no need to worry about entities that never came into existence, the claims of entities that will exist in the future do need to be considered in advance. It may be true, as Susan Okin puts it, that: "a human infant originates from a minute quantity of abundantly available and otherwise useless resources" (Okin, 1989, p 83). But these 'resources' have extraordinary potential. While an embryo has no thoughts, feelings or expectations, this is no reason not to take into account the fact that it might have future claims that could be affected even at this early stage. Again, new possibilities bring new ethical considerations and in this case, the ethical challenge is that there may well be a conflict between what some existing human beings want or appear to need and what another future person might be entitled to.

One thing in particular that a future person might be entitled to is knowledge of their own origins or, at a minimum, information about the special circumstances in which he or she came to be born. In a number of jurisdictions today, including New Zealand, parts of Australia and Sweden, legislation has been introduced to guarantee the right of people born from donated gametes to know the identity of their genetic parent. The UK will give this right to such children in the future, although it will not apply retrospectively. What seems to have been increasingly accepted is that, both ethically and legally, it is wrong to deprive a person of available records of their genetic origin and hence of their ancestry and other relationships. At a minimum, this argument can be made on medical grounds, as a result of new knowledge about genetics and illness, but many children, now adults, who were born by donation, have made a strong case for it, too, on social grounds.

## Genetic relations

A right to knowledge is one thing, but a right to be in touch with, or even brought up by, a genetically related person is more open to challenge. So, are children losing something valuable if their origins necessarily deprive them of a genetic link to their carers, especially if the relationship in question is that of a mother or a father? Single women and lesbian couples can, without too much difficulty, have access to sperm donation to have children and while this is often legally permitted as well as medically possible, the situation of single men and gay male couples is more complicated. It has been done, but it requires an egg donor and a surrogate to bear the child (the same woman could, of course, fulfil both functions). In both cases, however, organisations exist to meet the needs of same-sex couples by supplying gametes of the opposite sex.

But is there a right to found any sort of family? In some circumstances single women, single men and lesbian and gay couples can adopt children. Does it follow that people in all these categories should be able to create families of their own choosing? Many believe that there should be a right of equal access for all. But in opening the door to this possibility, the UK Parliament judged it necessary to add a legal requirement to the 1990 Human Fertilisation and Embryology Act that the need of a child for a father should be taken into account. Since that date, technology has developed to a stage where the need of a child for a mother cannot be taken for granted either. For the first time, it is necessary to ask if children have a right to a mother, a right to a father, or even a right to two parents one male, one female? This is a new and untrodden area for society.

While many western countries accept parity in law as far as adult same-sex unions are concerned, the involvement of children once again raises some additional considerations. Can two people of the same sex really substitute for a male and a female parent? This is not a question about purely practical possibilities; same-sex partners often have children from a previous heterosexual relationship and do continue to care for them very well. They can also adopt children, either singly or together. So where the new technologies are concerned, the question is not so much what is possible as what should be taken as a model. There is a historic conception of mother and father common to most human beings and to deprive someone of either must be a significant step. Would it be unlawful discrimination to recognise this? In 2002 the European Parliament published a report recommending that unmarried partnerships, both heterosexual and homosexual, should be given the same rights as marriage. It would seem that this must include a right to found a family, even if it does not necessarily include a right to be helped to do so.

The new perspective represented by many recent legislative moves reflects a sea-change in public and political opinion on these matters. However, the implications of gender equality are not always thought through to their logical conclusion. Absent fathers are not uncommon, but what about children, male or female, without mothers? The basic sentiment of sympathy for a motherless child, common to most societies, is hard to disregard. Nevertheless, where assisted reproduction is concerned, a substitute is provided in the form of a different mother or a different father, and their commitment to parenting is likely to be very strong. It is an important tenet of a free society that it is wrong to rule out social arrangements designed to satisfy people's strong desires where this involves no serious harm to others. The issue turns, then, on whether this deprivation is a serious harm. Given the speed of the new developments, it may still be too early to establish this. It is difficult to know at this stage, for example, how it would feel to have been deliberately denied the maternal relationship. It is too easy, too, to generalise from the case of children born after the death of their father as a result of factors outside either parent's control, to that of children born following the deliberate exclusion of a parent. Considerations like these could justify a slower pace of change and a more cautionary approach to the 'new families' ideology. As Jonathan Glover has observed: "The normal state for a child is to have one parent of each sex. It is surely right to be very cautious about tampering with something so fundamental" (Glover, 1989, p 59).

## Designing babies

Within the medical field, there are other uses of the new technologies that are often approached on a case-by-case basis. Their object is not normally to fulfil purely social choices, but to help people avoid the trauma some inherited conditions can bring within families. These other choices are made possible by using the techniques of fertility treatment, in particular IVF (in vitro fertilisation), to create a number of embryos and select among them in order to base a pregnancy on a more secure basis or to avoid risking the birth of a child with a serious inherited condition. This technique, known as PGD, can enable parents and their medical advisers to select an embryo of a particular sex, to select for or against a disability, or even to choose an embryo as a potential tissue or bone marrow donor for another family member.

These various possibilities raise a number of ethical questions. But first, it is important to correct some common misunderstandings of the term 'designer babies'. This is often thought to mean that the embryo's genetic structure has been altered to create a 'designer baby' in a positive sense, or that prospective parents have chosen children for characteristics like intelligence, sporting prowess or good looks. But these are complex characteristics involving a number of genes and if such a scenario is ever to be possible, it is a long way in the future. What is possible now is to use the new technologies of assisted reproduction to avoid an undesired medical outcome for a child, usually a genetic condition that can be inherited within a family. Since some well-known genetic conditions are sex-linked, this can often be done simply by selecting an embryo of the unaffected sex. Whether people should be allowed to select for sex other than medical reasons is a more controversial issue. Some regard state interference to prevent this as an infringement of personal liberty. Again, however, there are broader aspects to be considered. For example, in groups where there is a cultural preference for males, it could place pressure on women to use this difficult and possibly hazardous route to pregnancy. On the other hand, many people would be sympathetic to a couple's wish to 'balance' their family in the sense of having children of both sexes.

However, even if limited to avoiding a serious medical risk, PGD still arouses controversy. In particular, some of those representing people with disabilities believe that if you are trying to eliminate known health problems, this implies that people with those problems are less worthy of respect than other people. They would prefer to see a more positive approach to those conditions and more help for families coping with them.

Disability advocates could, however, take this further and seek to use the technology to select for a condition that is usually regarded as a handicap. Finally, the technology can be used to bring a child into the world for someone else's good or well-being. Two examples can be used to illustrate these last two possibilities, both of which are controversial in that they seem to involve using the technology for ends that are not primarily directed to considering the good of the future child at all, but to some other end.

## Choosing a deaf child

People who are deaf often share a friendly and supportive community life, hence some deaf people would prefer to have children who are also deaf and so will be able to become members of their own community. In a much-discussed case in the US, this wish led to a deaf woman successfully seeking a deaf sperm donor in the hope of having a child who would also be deaf. (In this case, a sperm donor was sought because the would-be mother was a lesbian with a female partner.) The ethical challenge here is that, no matter how happy the resulting child might appear to be later in life, it seems to have been deliberately chosen to have a life that would lack something that other human beings take for granted and which most people regard as of very high value.

## Choosing a saviour sibling

The background to the second example is that children suffering from certain rare inherited diseases may be helped by a blood or bone marrow transfusion from a suitable donor, ideally a sibling. Parents may understandably hope that one of their existing children could provide a tissue match and if this is not the case, they may decide to have another child in the hope that the new child will be compatible as a donor for the sick child. Science can now assist this choice and the procedure involved is relatively straightforward, given the widespread use of assisted reproduction. It involves producing a number of embryos, which can then be examined in vitro to see if there is an embryo free of the condition that could become a child who is an ideal tissue match for the existing child.

Compassionate though this might seem, the question is whether the donor child is being fairly treated. Both the child's welfare and the child's rights are involved, and it is doubtful whether either can be adequately protected in these circumstances. The hope is that all that will be needed is the new-born baby's cord blood. However, if the cord blood donation fails, the new child is destined for a possible lifetime of pressure to donate whatever its ailing older sibling might need in the future. This could include not only repeated donations of bone marrow, but even non-replaceable organs. Sometimes an imaginative work of fiction can make an ethical point more clearly than an academic argument and in *My sister's keeper* Jodi Picoult paints a compelling portrait of the dilemmas that could be faced by a child conceived in this way (Picoult, 2004). The child in this novel seeks out a lawyer to help her challenge her parents' right to make medical decisions on her behalf. The ethical challenge here is that, no matter how excellent their situation in other respects, the 'saviour sibling' is a child who has been created in order to be used for a purpose that goes beyond that child's own interests.

## Conclusions and contemporary challenges for new reproductive technologies

Some people believe that the whole process of reproduction has become over-medicalised. Others object to the aspect of 'playing God' that seems to be involved when life is created in these novel ways, particularly when an embryologist injects a sperm into a human egg, bringing into existence an embryo that can become a unique individual person. These are matters of continuing controversy, but reproductive possibilities do not end here and scientific developments continue to open up new and equally contentious frontiers for exploration. Most challenging of all is the fact that embryos can have other uses, including supplying stem cells for some dramatic new medical possibilities. One of these might be human cloning, but the idea of cloning human beings has made such an adverse impact on public opinion that many legislatures have moved quickly to ban it. There is, however, a distinction between reproductive and therapeutic cloning. Both use stem cell technology, but while the first seeks to produce a cloned human person, the second makes use of the early stage embryo in a quest for new approaches to illness. On the basis of this distinction, research using stem cell technology is going ahead on a legally accepted basis in many parts of the world.

In this chapter, the question has been raised in a number of different contexts of how far law should control developments in this area. Some people see regulation of genetic research and technology as based on essentially religious assumptions. While many of these issues are of concern to religious groups, they have a broad ethical dimension that is not dependent on a faith perspective. Indeed, one very widely accepted moral and political principle that applies here is the duty to protect the vulnerable. So, where it is intended that an embryo should become a human person, the vulnerability of that future person to the choices that are made at the embryonic stage deserves recognition. In deploying the new technologies, society has a responsibility to protect the welfare and rights of people at a stage of existence when they are unable to protect them for themselves. Adults' choices and wishes do matter. But there is also a child's perspective, when children created in new and unusual ways are deprived of many of the things that children born in the ordinary way are able to take for granted. This must include some careful thought about their rights as regards their own genetic relatives, their knowledge of their origins and their own likely future role and choices.

The UN General Assembly, in the 1997 Universal Declaration on the Human Genome and Human Rights, spoke of certain risks: one, the possible collapse of society's material and moral solidarity towards vulnerable people; another, a risk that the inequality of distribution of the benefits of research and its applications could jeopardise the principle of the equal dignity of individuals. Guarding against these risks continues to be the important ethical challenge posed by the new technologies of reproduction.

## References

Council of Europe (1950) 'The European Convention for the Protection of Human Rights and Fundamental Freedoms, 1950, together with its Protocols, as amended by Protocol No 11', in I. Brownlie and G.S. Goodwin-Gill (eds) (2002) *Basic documents on human rights* (4th edn), Oxford: Oxford University Press, pp 398-422.

Dworkin, R. (1993) *Life's dominion*, London: Harper Collins.

European Parliament (2002) *Report on the human rights situation in the European Union (2001)*, Committee on Citizens' Freedoms and Rights, Justice and Home Affairs, Joke Swiebel, rapporteur, A5-0451/2002.

Glover, J. (1989) *Fertility and the family*, London: Fourth Estate.

Harris, J. (1998) 'Rights and reproductive choice', in J. Harris and S. Holm (eds) *The future of human reproduction*, Oxford: Oxford University Press, pp 5-37.

Okin, S. (1989) *Justice, gender and the family*, New York, NY: Basic Books.

Picoult, J. (2004) *My sister's keeper*, London, Hodder.

Robertson, J.A. (1996) *Children of choice: Freedom and the new reproductive technologies*, Princeton, NJ: Princeton University Press.

Ryan, M.A. (1990) *The argument for unlimited procreative liberty*, Hastings Center Report, New York, NY: Hastings Centre Publications, pp 6-12.

UN (United Nations) (1948) 'Universal Declaration of Human Rights', in I. Brownlie and G.S. Goodwin-Gil (eds) (2002) *Basic documents on human rights* (4th edn), Oxford: Oxford University Press, pp 18-23.

UN (1997) 'Universal Declaration on the Human Genome and Human Rights', in I. Brownlie and G.S. Goodwin-Gill (eds) (2002) *Basic documents on human rights* (4th edn), Oxford: Oxford University Press, pp 810-16.

Warnock, M. (1985) *Question of life: The Warnock Report on human fertilisation and embryology*, Oxford: Blackwell.

# FIFTEEN

# Ethics: caring for children and young people

*David Hodgson*

## Summary

In this chapter, two cases involving children are used to illustrate problems and challenges in contemporary childcare practice. These cases also serve to highlight how, in focusing on individual circumstances, attention can be drawn away from broader ethical questions that may be relevant to the treatment of children. A similar tendency to overlook this broader perspective is noted from an overview of recent childcare reforms set out in *Every child matters* (DfES, 2003a). A historical and conceptual analysis of childcare discourse charts the interaction between ideas about children's relationships, interests and rights, concluding that the concept of 'children's rights' challenges some conventional ways of interpreting human experience. Insights from this analysis are used to explore four aspects of the reform agenda with a view to promoting respect for human rights in professional practice.

### Two young people

Victoria Climbié, an eight-year-old child from the Ivory Coast, lived in temporary accommodation with her great aunt and the aunt's boyfriend. After admission to hospital for suspected non-accidental injuries, Victoria was referred to social services but discharged to her aunt's care after two weeks. In the course of 11 months, Victoria became known to a further three social services departments, three housing authorities, two police child protection teams, a specialist centre managed by the NSPCC (National Society for the Prevention of Cruelty to Children) and was admitted to hospital again for medical problems associated with suspected deliberate harm. She was observed by several people, lay and professional, to be fearful and ill at ease with her 'carers', who adopted an authoritarian and punitive attitude towards her. Shortly after a third hospital admission, Victoria died of hypothermia in circumstances described by the pathologist as the worst case of deliberate harm to a child that he had ever seen. There were 128 separate injuries to her body.

Lela, a 12-year-old West African child, lived with her aunt and partner on a temporary residence order, having entered the country illegally with the aunt two years previously. Previous child protection investigations of neglect and physical punishment had been inconclusive, with Lela strongly hinting at, and then retracting, allegations. One day Lela asked a teacher if she could speak to someone in confidence about her feelings. A worker from the Child and Adolescent Mental Health Service (CAMHS) agreed to see her at school. Over subsequent months concerns gradually emerged about Lela's low mood, self-harm and routine neglect at home. Eventually, Lela allowed the CAMHS worker to set out detailed concerns about her situation to social services. Subsequently, she moved to live with foster carers, resumed her disrupted education, obtained exceptional leave to remain in the country and negotiated contact with her wider family.

In both of these cases, a child separated from her family of origin was physically and emotionally abused while living with extended kin in precarious material and legal circumstances. Whereas Lela found someone able to appreciate her predicament, no one saw or heard the extent of Victoria's distress. With professional help, Lela negotiated a situation of safety that enabled her to remain connected with her family and culture. In contrast, no meaningful communication with Victoria was established and no sustained attempts were made to give priority to her basic human rights.

In seeking explanations for Victoria's death and Lela's survival, our attention is inevitably drawn to comparisons between the two cases: for example, family and cultural background, the depth of the perpetrators' cruelty, the level of each child's vulnerability affected by age and circumstances, and the capabilities of the professionals involved. However, there is another level of analysis that seeks to understand how prevailing attitudes and values might influence perceptions of the problems facing children. This moral and political climate is likely to have a bearing on professional ethics in childcare. The chapter seeks to explore this broader ideological terrain in order to consider possible implications for the exercise of professional judgement in childcare cases.

A starting point for investigating ethical dimensions in childcare is the government Green Paper, *Every child matters* (DfES, 2003a). Arguably the most significant statement of childcare policy in recent years, the Green Paper presented proposals to reform children's services in the light of the Inquiry into Victoria's death (DH, 2003). Several of these proposals subsequently resulted in legal changes introduced by the 2004 Children Act.

## An overview of *Every child matters*

It is possible to distinguish three levels of problem analysis within the Green Paper that are briefly discussed here (Lymbery and Butler, 2004).

**Table 15.1:** Levels of problem analysis in childcare

| Macro | Mezzo | Micro |
|---|---|---|
| Socioeconomic and cultural factors | Child welfare system – organisational and bureaucratic factors | Individual interactions – children, families, professionals |

### *Socioeconomic and cultural factors (macro-level)*

The title of the document *Every child matters* suggests a concern for the principle of equity in childcare, an impression reinforced by the vision for achieving five outcomes for children's well-being (being healthy, staying safe, enjoying and achieving, making a positive contribution and economic well-being) through greater interagency cooperation. However, the Green Paper did not present an explicit moral agenda about the care of children, preferring to focus on apparently technical and organisational issues.

### *Child welfare system (mezzo-level)*

The most detailed problem analysis was reserved for child welfare systems. Referring to 12 missed opportunities to 'save' Victoria documented in the Inquiry, the Green Paper asserted that "social services, the police and the NHS failed ... to do the basic things well to protect her" (DfES, 2003b, p 5). 'Common threads' identified in reports into child deaths stretching back to the 1970s include "poor co-ordination; failure to share information; absence of anyone with a strong sense of accountability; and frontline workers trying to cope with staff vacancies, poor management and a lack of effective training" (DfES, 2003b, p 5).

Tighter structures for accountability and integration at local, regional and national level were promised, together with workforce reforms to enhance recruitment, training and leadership. Further proposals to improve communication and coordination in practice included legal and technical steps to overcome barriers to information sharing, a common assessment framework, co-located multidisciplinary teams and a named lead professional for all children known to more than one agency.

## Individual interactions (micro-level)

The Green Paper did not pose any particular moral or ethical questions in relation to the horrific abuse perpetrated on Victoria or the transient involvement of professionals in the case. For example, no opinion was ventured as to whether prevailing attitudes towards children might have contributed to events in the case. However, the authors were more forthcoming in relation to other moral problems, notably "truancy, anti-social behaviour and offending" (DfES, 2003b, p 9), for which targeted support was prescribed and, as a last resort, compulsory parenting orders for parents who condone such behaviour.

To summarise, this major policy statement did not place moral and ethical questions about the care of children or the judgement of professionals at the centre of the reform agenda. The rhetoric of *Every child matters* (DfES, 2003a) affirmed the value of childhood in a general sense, while lacking any analysis of current beliefs and attitudes. The judgement of professionals was presented as a problem to be managed by regulation.

## Childcare language: relationships, interests and rights

It is possible that the language of decision making may provide more insight into how underlying values can influence perceptions of childcare issues and problems. Three significant terms that feature in this discourse are 'relationships', 'interests' and 'rights' (Fox Harding, 1997). The following discussion suggests that 'children's relationships' and 'children's interests' are uncontested terms, whereas the language of 'children's rights' continues to provoke widespread anxiety. Much of this anxiety is focused on perceived tensions between the rights of parents and the responsibility of the state to promote improved standards of childcare. A brief analysis of ideas about rights, individualism and human value seeks to uncover historical explanations for this state of affairs and points towards alternative ways of conceptualising problems and solutions in childcare. These insights may enable us to consider aspects of the *Every child matters* reform agenda in a different light.

## Ideologies of human value

According to Lee (2005), current interpretations of the idea of 'rights' can be understood in the context of wider social and economic transformations that were accompanied by changes in the way value or worth is assigned to different groups of people. Drawing on the work of Taylor and Gutmann (1992), Lee (2005) draws attention to the gradual shift from strict hierarchies of medieval societies in which human value was determined by birth, connection and relationship (the principle of 'honour') towards industrialised societies that increasingly adopted the principle of 'dignity'. This principle signifies "the possession of, and what is owed to, each and every person regardless of the conditions of their birth" (Lee, 2005, p 23), namely equality of respect.

A means of rationing the distribution of this badge of 'dignity' was required that was consistent with the limited redistribution of economic, social and cultural possessions permitted by capitalism. Lee (2005) explains that this rationing mechanism was provided by the idea of 'level of development', a concept providing a pretext for colonial rule abroad as well as the maintenance of inequalities at home. The relevance for attitudes towards children becomes clearer when it is recognised that the present day understanding of childhood is predicated on assumptions about children as incomplete beings in need of development (Lee, 2001).

Within this ideological context, a very particular formulation of rights was adopted that was consistent with the ethos of a market economy. Rights (regarded as synonymous with 'interests') were defined as freedoms from state interference in private life and property. Rights holders were distinguished by their apparent independence and self-authorship, as befitting those who had attained an advanced 'level of development'. As a result, 'rights' came to be understood as being antithetical to 'relationships'. This exclusive version of rights is also associated with a particularly compartmentalised or dualistic view of human experience that maintains a strict separation between, for example, reason and emotion, objective and subjective experience, the self and the other, matters of private concern and public interest (Lukes, 1973).

For as long as 'level of development' was preserved as a mechanism for rationing the allocation of human value, it would be ideologically difficult to accord value to children. However, as industrialisation increasingly dictated the need for investment in children as the source of future productivity, a reconfiguration of ideas concerning the human value of children became necessary. The resulting reformulation provided the basis for an ethico-legal discourse that continues to exert an influence in present day childcare practice, some elements of which are described below.

## Children's relationships

Children's relationships, notably with parents or other primary carers, remain important as a source of their human value. The principle of honour survives to the extent that the law on parental responsibility still places children as parental possessions, although the possessory right of parents is increasingly justified as a freedom for all family members from interference by the state (Douglas, 2004). This freedom is articulated as the right to respect for private and family life, home and correspondence (Article 8, Schedule 1, 1998 Human Rights Act). Indeed, the courts have recently emphasised that "the mutual enjoyment by parent and child of each other's company constitutes a fundamental element of family life…" (R(G) v Barnet London Borough Council; R(W) v Lambeth London Council; R(A) v Lambeth London Borough Council [2003] UKHL 57, [2004] 1 FLR 454, at para 68 [per Lord Hope of Craighead], in Harris-Short, 2005, p 173), suggesting recognition of a reciprocal right of parents and children similar to that embodied in Scottish law (section 2, 1995 Children (Scotland) Act).

Tensions between the rights of parents and the rights of the state to intervene in parenting are a source of continuing debate (Archard, 2003). In public law, the principle of non-interference with parental discretion is supported by the notion that a threshold of 'significant harm' is required to justify compulsory action by professionals and the courts to safeguard children (Parts IV and V, 1989 Children Act). On the other hand, recent cases have highlighted concerns about the persistent failure of the courts, local authorities and childcare professionals to respect procedural and substantive rights owed to parents under the 1998 Human Rights Act (for example, Re G (Care:

*Challenge to Local Authority's Decision)* [2003] EWHC 551 (Fam), [2003] 2 FLR 42, in Harris-Short, 2005, p 170).

## Children's interests

It is arguable that the position of children is even less assured than that of their parents. The idea of 'children's interests', when detached from the concept of 'rights', has provided a rationale for investment in child welfare that does not demand acknowledgement of children as beings who are, in Lee's terms, "self-possessed" (Lee, 2001, p 46). The welfare principle (section 1, 1989 Children Act) appears to give priority to children without necessarily requiring undue attention to what children may be interested in. On the other hand, the welfare principle has also been criticised for giving insufficient priority to the interests and rights of parents, leading to advocacy of a relationship-based approach to child welfare decisions (Herring, 2005).

National and international statutes require decision makers to give due consideration to the child's viewpoint (sections 17, 20 and 47, 1989 Children Act, as amended; Article 12, 1989 United Nations [UN] Convention on the Rights of the Child). However, the child's capacity to make decisions is regarded as a matter of judgement, usually by those who also have discretion to define children's interests, such as parents, professionals and judges. Furthermore, even if judged to be competent, a child's refusal to consent to proposed interventions may be overridden (Fortin, 2003, ch 3).

## Children's rights

Discomfort with the language of children's rights emanates from several quarters. Harris-Short (2005) has argued that there is scepticism about using rights language in children's cases because jurisprudence is weighted in favour of parents rather than children. In contrast, other commentators have argued that the discourse of rights is conceptually inappropriate to account for the position of children and potentially damaging to their interests through its insensitivity to nurturing relationships on which children depend (Cooper, 1998; Arneil, 2002). Thus, the idea of children's rights can be portrayed as a weapon in an apparent struggle between the power of parents and the parenting power of the state, exercised by the courts and childcare professionals.

To summarise, in the allocation of human value to children, tensions between the conflicting principles of 'honour' and 'dignity' continue to be managed through an interplay between 'children's relationships' and 'children's interests'. Children's rights gain recognition when construed as interests to be defined in detail by adults but are otherwise criticised for undermining family relationships and parental rights. The autonomy of parents is emphasised in principle but not necessarily respected in practice.

In the light of the historical analysis of ideas about human value, it is possible to appreciate why the concept of children's rights has powerful potential to cause ideological disturbance. Little disruption is caused by children's rights that are defined as interests to be determined by adults. However, when advanced as a claim to more substantial recognition of dignity and self-possession for children, the concept of children's rights begins to challenge established ideas of human rights that are associated with the dualistic interpretation of human experience described earlier.

An alternative ethics of human rights begins to emerge that recognises interdependence alongside individuality. Instead of discounting children's rights, an attempt can be made to reframe human rights for children and adults within the context of childcare, acknowledging the centrality of relationships alongside the recognition that all people have distinct interests (Banks, 2006). The following discussion reconsiders some key aspects of the current reform agenda with a view to clarifying the implications for professionals of respecting human rights in childcare practice.

## *Every child matters:* universal rights and professional judgements

Four aspects of the *Every child matters* reform programme are explored here. In the first case, questions about definitions of child abuse and the boundaries of personal integrity are subjected to scrutiny. The second aspect is concerned with the representation of children's voices in policy and practice. The third example highlights tensions between the obligation to provide support for families and the responsibility to safeguard children. Finally, some ideas about competence and the capacity for decision making are examined.

## Definitions of abuse and personal integrity

### Physical and emotional harm

Respect for personal integrity depends on the observance of rules concerning physical and mental boundaries. Article 3 of the European Convention on Human Rights states "no one shall be subjected to torture or to inhuman or degrading treatment or punishment", such as the physical and mental harms suffered by Victoria and Lela.

Surprisingly, neither the Victoria Climbié Inquiry Report nor the Green Paper (DfES, 2003a) scrutinised the substance of civil or criminal law in relation to child abuse. A chapter of the report about the detrimental impact of assumptions linked to 'race' and culture omitted to make a connection with the broader legal and cultural prejudice against state 'interference' in child rearing (DH, 2003, ch 16).

Apparently anxious to avoid encroaching on parental discretion, the government resisted a cross–party attempt to remove the defence of 'reasonable chastisement' for parents or carers who face prosecution for criminal assault (section 1, 1933 Children and Young Persons Act). A compromise amendment retained the defence for common assault on children (section 58, 2004 Children Act), a provision that could be used to defend parents in cases of emotional harm or assaults in which no physical mark is evident (Lyon, 2003; Newell, 2005). Consequently, the group considered most vulnerable to abuse remain disadvantaged in a highly symbolic area of law, contrary to the spirit and, arguably, the letter of human rights legislation (Schedule 1, Article 14, 1998 Human Rights Act).

### Information and personal integrity

Reform proposals to improve information sharing among childcare professionals highlighted further questions about personal boundaries related to privacy. It is possible that children will be disadvantaged as a group when not perceived as having 'ownership' of personal information.

The 2004 Children Act provides for the establishment of personal information databases about children with the dual purpose of facilitating "early, coherent, intervention" and assisting "service planning" (2004 Children Act, Explanatory Notes, para 70). The new measure lists people and agencies that can be required to disclose information and those permitted to disclose, notwithstanding the duty of confidence (1998 Data Protection Act). This reform seeks to overcome barriers to interprofessional communication but could jeopardise an ethic of confidentiality valued by young people such as Lela.

The debate about this measure highlighted tensions between professional groups seeking to preserve their discretion to decide on matters of confidentiality and disclosure (Taylor, 2005). Subsequent draft guidance appeared to play up these tensions by proposing to treat health professionals as a special case requiring a unique procedure to preserve the confidential relationship as far as possible (DfES, 2005). The overall effect of the guidance may be to lower the threshold at which confidential information can be disclosed without the child's consent (Hamilton, 2005).

Alternatively, if child protection was reframed so as to give greater prominence to children's rights to privacy, childcare professionals might feel more encouraged in giving priority to practices that promote mutual respect in relation to information sharing, including respect for children's concerns about confidentiality and loss of control over the sharing of information (Featherstone and Evans, 2004).

## Representation of children's voices

Alongside skills for involving young people in negotiations about privacy and personal disclosure, there is an important role for professionals to promote children's voices in policy and practice decisions, as highlighted in Lela's experience. The idea of independent advocacy for children has gained ground in law and policy over recent years, although there is still debate over the legitimacy of this activity (Dalrymple, 2003). Whether recent reforms will enhance or undermine the representation of children's views remains to be seen. The creation of a Children's Commissioner for England in 2005 acknowledged the need for an independent national voice for children. However, this mechanism has been criticised for falling short of international standards, with independent powers of inquiry and investigation heavily circumscribed (Newell, 2005).

As for the explicit objectives of the reform agenda, the five statutory outcomes for measuring children's well-being (Section 10, 2004 Children Act) apparently derived from consultations about what "mattered most to children and young people" (DfES, 2003b, p 7). However, subtle changes in the wording of these outcomes during the legislative process signified that paternalistic notions of 'children's interests' would be preserved (for example, 'being safe' was expressed as 'protection from harm and neglect'). A subsequent consultation with young people sponsored by the Commission for Social Care Inspection found that, while the children consulted were happy to agree with the statutory outcomes, seven more were requested to make a "Children's Dozen". The list included "family; friends; enough food and drink; fun; love; respect and being happy" (Social Services Parliamentary Monitor, 2005, p 13). This broader vision seems to emphasise the achievement of rights through relationships. Childcare professionals make a significant contribution to overcoming tokenism in the representation of children's views, firstly, by careful analysis of the factors that influence their assessments of the child's welfare and, secondly, by recognising circumstances in which independent advocacy for children is required.

## Safeguarding children and supporting families

A recurring theme in childcare policy and practice is the tension between the objectives of protecting children and enabling them to remain with their families (Parton, 1997). The earlier discussion of childcare discourses underlined that professionals have a responsibility to protect children from abuse while having regard for the privacy and family life of both parents and children (Schedule 1, Article 8, 1998 Human Rights Act). *Every child matters* (DfES, 2003a) represents the latest in a series of attempts to shift the emphasis from reactive to preventive child welfare services (DH, 1995).

Child protection studies (Munro, 2002; Gardner, 2005) and research evidence linking child health outcomes with structural inequalities (Jack, 2004) indicate that family support is crucial for safeguarding children. If more children and parents are to be spared the damaging impact of permanent family separation through skilled interventions supported by material help, legal and policy frameworks will need to be more sympathetic to the ethics of support for families.

According to Fawcett et al (2004), contemporary child and family policies are rooted in the idea of the 'social investment state', a 'New Deal' for state investment in individuals on the basis of their value as potentially productive 'human capital'. The ethos of the social investment state accentuates personal responsibility and downplays the impact of socioeconomic circumstances. As a result, historical distinctions between the 'deserving' and 'undeserving' tend to resurface as part of the process of rationing scarce resources (Jordan, 2000; Hendrick, 2003). Moral judgements of this kind will continue to colour professional discretion while poverty remains a central problem for families who come to the attention of childcare agencies (Preston,

2005). Recent legal changes appear to involve a further shift away from entitlement towards discretionary allocation of family support services, for example, those highlighted by Masson (2003), in connection with policies to increase the adoption of children in care (2002 Adoption and Children Act). In the midst of this moral climate, a greater onus is placed on childcare professionals to counteract discriminatory judgements that might lead to the withdrawal of support services for poorer families.

## Personal and professional competence

The foregoing discussion has raised ethical questions about decision-making competence among children, parents and professionals, for example, Lela's capacity to negotiate the kind of support she required; the ability of parents to make decisions in their children's interests; and the capability of professionals to reach measured judgements about interventions with families. Forms of competence vary but common themes may emerge from a broader reappraisal of this issue.

Several commentators (for example, Jones, 2004; Munro, 2004) have sought to understand the nature and depth of apparent incompetence reported to the Victoria Climbié Inquiry. Two aspects of competence were notably absent: firstly, a competence of reason, to do "relatively straightforward things well" (DH, 2003, para 1.66); secondly, a competence of feeling, to demonstrate emotional empathy and intuitive understanding to appreciate the oppressive impact of Victoria's plight.

Munro (2004) observes that the Inquiry, like previous ones, concentrated on findings of human fallibility, resulting in recommendations for increased regulation and diminished professional discretion. An alternative emphasis is suggested that focuses on system characteristics and forms of 'local rationality' with a tendency to generate specific kinds of human error. According to Munro (2004, p 385), the culture of managerialism in social work organisations can actually discourage 'emotional wisdom' by downgrading feelings and reframing social work tasks as 'essentially cognitive'. The mechanical use of assessment tools and rigid implementation of targets or performance indicators may also contribute to emotional detachment from children and their families. Overall, this analysis suggests that reform measures designed to reduce the scope for logical error may further impede the development of 'mindful' childcare practice that combines reason and intuition (Jones, 2004).

Conditions conducive to sound professional practice might be articulated more clearly if competence was regarded more as a product of association than separation – of reason and emotion, of objective criteria and subjective context, of interdependence rather than isolated independence. Time, skill and relationships could more readily be directed towards the goal of enhancing the sense of self-authorship and continuity of being in children and adults (Bell, 2002). This perspective raises questions about competence and incompetence among children, parents and practitioners. Consequently, there may be a greater recognition of how power can affect judgements and decisions (Houston, 2003). Other health and social care commentators have explored this unorthodox view of competence, for example, in relation to the refusal of psychiatric treatment (Shaw, 2002) and elective surgery (Daniel et al, 2005).

## Conclusions and contemporary challenges in caring for children and young people

This chapter began by describing how the perception of problems associated with current childcare practice can be skewed towards a focus on distinctions at the level of individual cases and away from broader moral and political issues: specifically, prevailing values associated with childhood. Insights from a brief conceptual and historical analysis of childcare discourse helped to identify ethical challenges arising from four aspects of the *Every child matters* reforms: firstly, advocating children's equal rights to physical and emotional integrity, recognising that personal privacy is central to child protection; secondly, maximising formal and informal structures for representation of young people's perspectives; thirdly, challenging contradictions in law and policy that detract from family support, fuel judgemental attitudes and erode professional creativity; and, finally, using skill and judgement to pursue models of competence building with children, families and fellow professionals.

### Acknowledgements
I would like to thank colleagues in the Faculty of Health and Social Care Sciences, Kingston University and St George's University of London for advice on this chapter: Nigel Elliott, Principal Lecturer in Social Work; Teresa Horgan, Senior Lecturer in Physiotherapy; Linda King, Principal Lecturer in Physiotherapy; Robert Stanley, Senior Lecturer in Ethics; and Professor Olive Stevenson, Visiting Professor of Social Work. I would also like to thank Deborah Bowman, Senior Lecturer in Medical Ethics and Law, St George's University of London; Jane Dalrymple, Senior Lecturer, Faculty of Health and Social Care,

University of the West of England; Nicola Moxham, Approved Social Worker; and Sharon Start, Independent Psychotherapist.

## References

Archard, D. (2003) *Children, family and the state*, Aldershot: Ashgate.

Arneil, B. (2002) 'Becoming versus being: a critical analysis of the child in liberal theory', in D. Archard and C. Macleod (eds) *The moral and political status of children*, Oxford: Oxford University Press, ch 5.

Banks, S. (2006) *Ethics and values in social work* (3rd edn), Basingstoke: Palgrave Macmillan.

Bell, M. (2002) 'Promoting children's rights through the use of relationship', *Child and Family Social Work*, vol 7, pp 1-11.

Cooper, D. (1998) 'More law and more rights: will children benefit?', *Child and Family Social Work*, vol 3, no 2, pp 77-86.

Dalrymple, J. (2003) 'Professional advocacy as a force for resistance in child welfare', *British Journal of Social Work*, vol 33, no 8, pp 1043-62.

Daniel, E., Kent, G., Binney, V. and Pagdin, J. (2005) 'Trying to do my best as a mother: decision-making in families of children undergoing elective surgical treatment for short stature', *British Journal of Health Psychology*, vol 10, pp 101-14.

DfES (Department for Education and Skills) (2003a) *Every child matters*, Green Paper, Cm 5860, London: The Stationery Office.

DfES (2003b) *Every child matters: Summary* (available at www.everychildmatters.gov.uk/_files/ B889EFF62F56A9E4C69778A869B3DA44.pdf, accessed 14/8/05).

DfES (2005) *Consultation: Cross government guidance – Sharing information on children and young people* (available at www.dfes.gov.uk/consultations/downloadableDocs/Cross-GovGuidance%20v8%203%2008Nov05.pdf, accessed 8/02/06).

DH (Department of Health) (1995) *Child protection: Messages from research*, London: Social Research Unit, HMSO.

DH (2003) *The Victoria Climbié Inquiry*, London: DH.

Douglas, G. (2004) *An introduction to family law* (2nd edn), Oxford: Oxford University Press.

Fawcett, B., Featherstone, B. and Goddard, J. (2004) *Contemporary child care policy and practice*, Basingstoke: Macmillan.

Featherstone, B. and Evans, H. (2004) *Children experiencing maltreatment: Who do they turn to?*, London: NSPCC.

Fortin, J. (2003) *Children's rights and the developing law* (2nd edn), London: LexisNexis UK.

Fox Harding, L. (1997) *Perspectives in child care policy* (2nd edn), London: Longman.

Gardner, R. (2005) *Supporting families: Child protection in the community*, Chichester: Wiley.

Hamilton, C. (2005) 'Information sharing', *Childright*, vol 221, pp 3-5.

Harris-Short, S. (2005) 'Family law and the Human Rights Act 1998: judicial restraint or revolution?', *Child and Family Law Quarterly*, vol 17, no 3, pp 329-62.

Hendrick, H. (2003) *Child welfare: Historical dimensions, contemporary debate*, Bristol: The Policy Press.

Herring, J. (2005) 'Farewell welfare?', *Journal of Social Welfare and Family Law*, vol 27, no 2, pp 159-71.

Houston, S. (2003) 'Moral consciousness and decision-making in child and family social work', *Adoption & Fostering*, vol 27, no 3, pp 61-70.

Jack, G. (2004) 'Child protection at the community level', *Child Abuse Review*, vol 13, pp 368-83.

Jones, J. (2004) 'What being mindful really means in practice', *Childright*, no 194, pp 3-4.

Jordan, B. (2000) *Social work and the third way: Tough love as social policy*, London: Sage Publications.

Lee, N. (2001) *Childhood and society: Growing up in an age of uncertainty*, Buckingham: Open University Press.

Lee, N. (2005) *Childhood and human value: Development, separation and separability*, Maidenhead: Open University Press.

Lukes, S. (1973) *Individualism*, Oxford: Basil Blackwell.

Lymbery, M. and Butler, S. (eds) (2004) *Social work ideals and practice realities*, Basingstoke: Palgrave Macmillan.

Lyon, C. (2003) *Child abuse* (3rd edn), Bristol: Family Law (Jordan Publishing Ltd).

Masson, J. (2003) 'The impact of the Adoption and Children Act 2002 – Part 2', *Family Law*, September, pp 644-9.

Munro, E. (2002) *Effective child protection*, London: Sage Publications.

Munro, E. (2004) 'Improving practice: child protection as a systems problem', *Child and Youth Services Review*, vol 27, pp 375-91.

Newell, P. (2005) 'Education and Skills Memoranda' (available at www.publications.parliament.uk/pa/cm200405/cmselect/cmeduski/uc40-iv/40m01.htm, accessed 15/10/05).

Parton, N. (ed) (1997) *Child protection and family support*, London: Routledge.

Preston, G. (ed) (2005) *At greatest risk: The children most likely to be poor*, London: CPAG.

Shaw, M. (2002) 'When young people refuse treatment: balancing autonomy and protection', in Rt Hon L.J. Thorpe and C. Cowton (eds) *Delight and dole – The Children Act 10 years on*, Bristol: Family Law (Jordan Publishing Ltd).

Social Services Parliamentary Monitor (2005) 'Children agree to being healthy and staying safe', *Cadmus Newsletters*, No 150, 29 August, Croydon, p 13.

Taylor, A. (2005) 'Demand for practitioners in sensitive work to be left off databases', *Community Care*, Sutton: Reed Business Publishing, 27 January–2 February, p 12.

Taylor, C. and Gutmann, A. (1992) *Multiculturalism and the politics of recognition*, Princeton, NJ: Princeton University Press, in N. Lee (2005) *Childhood and human value: Development, separation and separability*, Maidenhead: Open University Press.

# SIXTEEN

# Ethical dilemmas in caring for people with complex disabilities

*Keith Andrews*

## Summary

Complex disabilities, usually of a neurological cause, result in a combination of physical, cognitive and behavioural disorders. The disabilities not only affect the individual but also the family and to some extent society. The impact of these disabilities creates a range of ethical dilemmas in the areas of confidentiality; decision making for those who lack mental capacity; advance statements; decisions about withholding or withdrawing treatment; and involvement of people with disabilities in teaching and publications. All of these factors have an impact on professional and informal carers, while creating a challenge for statutory bodies in their responsibilities towards people with disabilities. Although these dilemmas may be difficult to resolve, there are certain ethical principles that can help in the decision making and caring process.

## Introduction

Complex disabilities are usually due to neurological disorders, especially those affecting the brain. The disabilities are complex in that they are a combination of impairments affecting motor, sensory, cognitive, behavioural and social functioning. Ethical principles of beneficence, non-maleficence, autonomy and justice all play a part in decision making in complex disabilities but are not straightforward (Beauchamp and Childress, 2001). Ethical decisions will largely be influenced by whether or not the person has the capacity to make decisions and whether the condition they have is static or deteriorating.

## Lack of mental capacity

The principle that a person must be assumed to have capacity unless otherwise proven is one of the main bases of the 2005 Mental Capacity Act (DCA, 2005). Any question of 'does this person lack mental capacity?', however, requires the retort 'for what?'. Global lack of capacity is rare, except in the vegetative/minimally conscious states and possibly late stage dementia. A person may have capacity to decide which jumper to wear but not whether to have medical treatment; to decide whether to listen to music but not whether they need a bath; or to understand that they need treatment but not the implications of taking part in a research study. There is also the difficulty that mental capacity may fluctuate from day to day or hour to hour.

Fundamental principles are that the patient must understand what the medical treatment is; that somebody says it is needed; why the treatment is proposed; in broad terms the nature of the proposed treatment; the principal benefits and risks; and the consequences of not receiving the proposed treatment. Another fundamental principle is that the individual must be given every opportunity to make decisions. There are many factors that influence a person's ability to demonstrate capacity in decision making, including anxiety, medication, time of day, location, distractions such as background noise, the complex language used by clinicians and communication/linguistic problems. Thus, assessment may require the assistance of family members, a speech and language therapist, communication aids, pictures or other aids. The decision that someone lacks capacity therefore requires great skill, perseverance and discussion. Even where the person lacks capacity for the decision this does not give the right for others to make whatever decisions they like. There are two fundamental concepts, that the decision must be in the best interest of the person and that the least restrictive decision should be made.

## Best interests

'Best interest' is a difficult concept and one that causes considerable confusion and concern; it is not just what others believe is 'best' for the person. It is essential to try and find out, usually in discussion with family members and others who know the person, whether the person had previously expressed any views on the decision to be made, whether they had any beliefs or values that are likely to influence the decision if they had capacity and any other factors that they would be likely to consider if they were able to do so (2005 Mental Capacity Act). There is a general view (BMA, 2001; GMC, 2002) that while clinicians have to protect the health of their patients, this is limited to where there is a net benefit to the patient. If treatment fails, or ceases to be of benefit, then the justification for that treatment ceases. However, there are difficulties in withdrawing treatment once it has been started, rather than withholding treatment in the first place.

'Net benefit' is also a difficult concept. Medicine is concerned with benefits such as improving or maintaining health and quality of life. In doing so, it has to balance these against the side effects, burdens, tolerability and risks of the treatment; there is therefore a considerable amount of subjective judgement involved. The problem in the case of the person who does not have mental capacity is whether benefits of treatments outweigh the burdens of that treatment. The General Medical Council (2002, p 8) acknowledges that the "benefits and burdens for the patient are not always limited to purely medical considerations ... and doctors must not simply substitute their own values or those of the people consulted". Thus, it is not sufficient to make a decision purely on the medical benefit of treatment, but it is also necessary to take into account what the person's wishes would probably have been.

One of the problems is that there is a difference between making treatment decisions and making value-of-life decisions. While clinicians are qualified to make decisions about which treatment is worthwhile and which is not, they are no better qualified than the man in the street to decide which life is worthwhile and which is not. What is more, medicine is changing. Its transition from acute to chronic disease is prompting a transition from primarily objective to primarily subjective evidence of health and health care effectiveness (Sullivan, 2003). Thus, medical decision making is changing to focus on patients' lives rather than patients' bodies; this creates an emphasis in chronic disability on quality of life, as much as what is medically appropriate.

There is, however, the problem of our interpretation of what can be considered a good quality of life for the patient. Substituted judgement has problems in that it is not certain as to whether the person making the substituted judgement is influenced by their own personal beliefs rather than those of the patient. For example, in a study comparing the views of chronically ill, older people and those of their physicians, the physicians generally considered their older outpatients' quality of life to be worse than did the patients (Uhlmann and Pearlman, 1991). Similarly, physicians' opinion of the quality of life of ventilated people has been shown to underestimate the patient's own perception of quality of life (Bach et al, 1991). It is not only health professionals who underestimate quality of life. In a study by Menzel et al (2002), chronically ill and disabled patients generally rated the value of their lives in a given health state more highly than did other people imagining themselves to be in such states.

## Futility

One aspect of best interests is whether treatment is futile or not. There are several basic principles to futility of treatment, for instance, that the treatment is having no benefit or desirable effect; that it is having some benefit but the side effects are too damaging; or that although the treatment is having benefit, another condition makes it pointless. This concept of futility causes great problems for clinical staff. Hainsworth (1998) identified seven themes of concern from nurses dealing with patients with severe brain damage: fear and vulnerability, trying to connect (with patients), empathy, futility, feeling abused (by families), struggling for support (from colleagues and physicians) and seeking affirmation through physical care.

However, the issue is often not so much the futility of treatment but whether the life itself is futile. The concept of futility of a life is much more difficult. So much depends on the individual's religious and cultural upbringing, their education, values, beliefs and personal philosophy. Factors that might make someone decide that life was futile include uncontrollable pain, uncontrollable severe distress (for example, nausea), uncontrollable depression, no awareness of environment, awareness of the profundity of the disability, or some patients just have a wish to die.

## Least restriction

The second concept for decision making is that of least restriction. There is a dilemma in trying to get the right balance between the right for personal freedom and the duty of care. Spittle (1992), for instance, has argued that a case can be made for weak paternalistic interventions. The concept of least restriction means that any decision we make on behalf of a person lacking mental capacity is the least invasive of their function. For instance, rather than ban a confused person from the bathroom because they are at risk of scalding themselves, the least restrictive option would be to put temperature control valves on the taps to ensure that the water is not hot enough to scald (2004 Mental Capacity Bill Code of Practice, see DH, 2004).

## Autonomy in decision making

Simonds (2003) has pointed out that the simple principles of beneficence and non-maleficence have been augmented and sometimes challenged by a rising awareness of patient/consumer rights, and the public's expectation of greater involvement in medical, social and scientific affairs that affect them. He also points out that in a publicly funded health care system in which rationing (explicit or otherwise) is inevitable, the additional concepts of utility and distributive justice can easily come into conflict with the individual's right to autonomy.

## Advance decisions

Autonomy is extremely limited, if not impossible, for those individuals who lack the mental capacity to make decisions. For this reason the concept of advance decisions (sometime known as living wills) has come into the equation. Legally, from 2007, advance decisions become rules with clear safeguards (2005 Mental Capacity Act). These ensure that people may make a decision in advance to refuse treatment if they should lose capacity in the future. It is made clear in the Act that an advance decision will have no application to any treatment that a doctor considers necessary to sustain life unless the decision is in writing, signed and witnessed. In addition, there must be an express statement that the decision stands 'even if life is at risk'.

Clinicians may be asked to advise a person with disabilities about advance decisions. Inevitably there are pros and cons in writing an advance decision. On the one hand, the advance decision provides the individual with the opportunity to have a say in what happens to them should they become unable to make their own decisions. Secondly, it gives guidance, indeed instruction, to the clinician. Thirdly, it saves the family from the guilt involved in making decisions. On the other hand, advance statements are often unclear about situations under which they apply; there is often a lack of knowledge in the advice that is given; there is no opportunity to discuss the situation at the time, which might influence a change of mind of the patient; and it does not take into account any new developments. The latter point is covered in the 2005 Mental Capacity Act, in that a clinician must consider whether there are any new facts, that, if the patient had been aware of them, may have altered the decision.

## End of life decisions

Decision making is usually relatively straightforward when discussing the situation of someone who has severe neurological disability and is mentally competent to make decisions. Such people obviously have the right to make the decision as to what happens to them. Actually, this is only partly true because we can only refuse treatment, not insist on having it. Autonomy is, therefore, only partial. There is also a dilemma in that clinicians have a duty of care, which may conflict with the wishes of the patient. The difficulty is knowing where to draw the line.

Let us take two real examples that on the surface are seeking the same decision. First is Miss B, a tetraplegic lady on a ventilator following a brainstem haemorrhage (White and Baldwin, 2002). She communicated that she wanted the ventilator switched off. This created quite a dilemma for the clinical team. Here was a lady who was fully mentally competent, in a stable condition and yet wanted the doctors to end her life. The court upheld her right to refuse treatment (the ventilator), the ventilator was switched off and she died.

At around the same time, Dianne Pretty, a lady in the late stages of motor neurone disease, also wanted to end her life (Morris, 2003; Pedain, 2003; Cowley, 2004). She realised that she only had a short time to live and faced the prospect of a humiliating and distressing death. She was supported by her husband in wanting to be able to take steps to bring her life to a peaceful end at a time of her choosing. However, the decisions of the High Court, the Court of Appeal and the European Court were that her request be refused. The main argument being that this would be assisted suicide, and, while suicide has not been illegal since 1961, assisting suicide remains a crime.

Many people find this confusing. Here were two ladies who were mentally alert, both of whom wished to end their lives. One who was in a stable condition was allowed to die; the other with a terminal illness was not allowed to have her life ended at the time she wished. Had she had the physical ability to commit suicide it would have been legal, but to have aids or help provided to achieve this was illegal. In both cases it required someone to take an action, in one case by switching off the ventilator, in the other by providing a drug. In one case it was refusal of treatment, in the other assisted suicide. Some would argue that switching off the ventilator was assisting Miss B to commit suicide.

## Withholding versus withdrawing treatment

Another situation where there is debate about the end of life situation is in the decision to withhold or withdraw treatment, the most extreme being the withdrawal of nutrition and hydration from a person in a vegetative state. In clinical practice it seems easier not to start a treatment rather than having to consider withdrawing it at a later date. The difficulty here is that those who withhold treatment are not giving the patient the opportunity to recover, while those who decide to withdraw treatment have given the patient an opportunity to recover and only stopped the treatment when it was ineffective. This is particularly relevant in the case of the vegetative state where, in England and Wales, it is a requirement to seek a directive from the court to withdraw treatment but not to withhold it (*Airedale NHS Trust v Bland* [1993] 1 All ER 821). For this reason the decision-making process for whether to withhold treatment should be exactly the same as for withdrawing treatment, that is, the decisions should be made using the same criteria (BMA, 2001). The British Medical Association suggested that there should be greater emphasis placed on the reasons for providing the treatment rather than the justification for withholding it. They also were very clear that "treatment should never be withheld, when there is a possibility that it will benefit the patient, simply because withholding is considered to be easier than withdrawing treatment" (BMA, 2001, p 11).

## Best interests of withdrawal of nutrition and hydration

One of the most difficult ethical decisions in complex disability is how to respond to a request to withdraw nutrition and hydration from a profoundly brain damaged person. The principles discussed above are fine, but they do not actually tell us how to make a decision on best interests. Where the treatment is not benefiting the patient, then the treatment is not in their best interest. However, nutrition and hydration is obviously having the effect that is intended – providing maintenance of the integrity of healthy tissues. The difficulty is whether it is benefiting the patient in the broader sense that it cannot achieve consciousness or any return of the 'person'.

All of the requirements of best interests discussed above apply. The main discussion then revolves around the futility of treatment or probably more relevantly around the futility of the life of the person. There are several arguments used for not withdrawing nutrition and hydration. One is that all life is worth having, proposed by Vitalist Theory (Mariner, 1995; Keown, 1997; Mayo and Gunderson, 2002). Secondly, we cannot know that there is no 'awareness'. There is some support for this in a number of papers (Tresch et al, 1991; Childs et al, 1993; Andrews et al, 1996) describing misdiagnosis of the vegetative state as high as 42%. Thirdly, concerns exist that there are at least a small number of reports of people emerging from the vegetative state many years after the brain damage. Finally, there is always concern that there may be some new medical breakthrough that will enable the person to emerge.

On the other hand there are those who argue that since the vegetative person has no cognitive awareness the person has no interests in living. Other arguments include that it is an assault or battery on the individual to be inserting tubes without their consent; that there are very few people who would want to live in such a condition; that the chances of emergence are so slim as to make it unwarranted to keep all vegetative people alive; that the family are unable to grieve; and that there would be a more appropriate use of scarce resources.

## 'Do not attempt resuscitation' orders

One of the common decisions to be made is whether to attempt to resuscitate someone who has severe disabilities should they have a cardiopulmonary arrest. These are often known as 'do not resuscitate', or more accurately, 'do not attempt resuscitation' (DNAR) orders. Considerable concern has been expressed about the placement of DNAR statements in a clinical record without the agreement of the disabled, usually elderly, person (Levin et al, 1998; Ebrahim, 2000). Even if there is discussion, information given is often not recalled, viewpoints often change as the disease progresses (or regresses) and decisions are poorly understood (Sayers et al, 1997; Krumholz et al, 1998).

It could be argued that health care professionals have a responsibility to offer only those life-sustaining efforts that have a reasonable chance of being beneficial (Weber and Campbell, 1996). Even where the patient is involved in the decision there are considerable problems in deciding what to advise. Mohr and Kettler (1997) argue that the basic principle is the moral rule that the victim of a cardiac arrest has the right to survive and to receive cardiopulmonary resuscitation. The principle of beneficence is based on the fact that some patients do have their lives saved. However, resuscitative efforts still remain unsuccessful in the majority of cases, thus involving the principle of non-maleficence.

There is potential harm in that survivors may recover cardiac function, but sustain further severe hypoxic brain damage, thus leading to the concept of futility.

Whereas the mentally competent person has the right to decide that there should be a DNAR policy, this is obviously not applicable to the person who lacks capacity. In view of the fact that most people cannot be resuscitated and given the high risk of further damage to the brain, many people consider attempts to resuscitate as being unnecessarily interventional, with a higher risk of maleficence than beneficence. Many relatives agree with this approach, feeling that the patient would not have wanted resuscitation in the presence of such devastating brain damage. Other relatives argue that since the alternative to resuscitation is almost certain death, then everything should be done to keep the person alive. This is often the case where the relative is having difficulty in coming to terms with poor prognosis of the brain damage. There is then the ethical difficulty of doing what one thinks is right for the patient while 'damaging' the needs of the relative – or vice versa. While it is not appropriate to treat one person to benefit another person, it is doubtful whether the patient would have wanted their relative to be distressed unnecessarily. Some would argue that this is more a case of helping the relative to come to terms than for inappropriately treating the patient.

While most authorities fight shy of discussion about the resource implications of treatment, this is something that should not be avoided. Madl et al (1996) argue that efforts should be made to identify those with a poor prognosis on Intensive Care Units to ensure the appropriate use of resources. Mohr and Kettler (1997) argue that the principle of justice affects priorities in the allocation of health care resources. The decision made for a particular patient might delay or prevent emergency treatment in other patients who could receive greater benefit.

## Making recordings of people lacking mental capacity

Recordings, whether photographic, audio or video, may be requested in a number of circumstances including for direct clinical purposes (for example, to measure or demonstrate the effect of treatment); for indirect clinical purposes (for example, records for teaching, audit, research or publication in professional journals); or for non-clinical purposes (for example, for publicity, fundraising or media purposes). In making decisions about the use of such recordings a number of needs have to be met:

- the need to protect the autonomy and privacy of people with disabilities;
- the need to benefit patients by the use of modern recording technology to assist the clinical team provide optimal management;
- the need to train clinicians and others in the management of complex neurological disability;
- the need for the organisation to publicise its services so that clinicians will be aware of what is available for referral purposes;
- the need for the organisation to raise funds to benefit patients and residents;
- the need to educate the general public.

The decision about whether the recording can be made is relatively simple in the case of a person who has the capacity to understand the purpose for the recording. As long as the person agrees to the recording and the purpose for which it is to be used then the recording can be made. However, the decision is much more complicated in the case of the person who lacks the capacity to understand the purpose of the recording.

The main consideration is that every person has the right to expect that information about him or her will be treated as confidential. The basic principle for whether a recording is appropriate is that of best interest. A number of factors should be addressed, including:

- the patient's own wishes and values, including any advance statement. These are generally unavailable;
- where there is more than one option for making the recording, the option that is least restrictive of the patient's future choices should be used – this includes limiting the detail recorded, avoidance of any feature that identifies the patient and the use of other means of producing the required information;
- the views of people close to the patient, especially close relatives, partners, carers or proxy decision makers, about what opinion the patient is likely to have held about the recordings;
- any knowledge of the patient's religious, cultural and other non-medical views that might have an impact on the patient's wishes.

In general, recordings for direct clinical purposes are acceptable. Particular attention should be paid to ensure that privacy and dignity are maintained in any recording taken. Recordings should only be taken if the recording is important as a record of the clinical state of the patient; if it is important in showing the change over time of a particular clinical feature or features; or the recording is required to demonstrate the treatment or clinical management programme to be carried out. The minimum number of recordings required to achieve the stated objective should be used and any recordings not required to meet the stated objective must be destroyed. The recordings should, like any other part of the clinical records, only be shown to others on a need to know basis. The recordings are not to be used for any other purpose unless the appropriate procedure, described below, has been carried out.

Recordings for indirect clinical use, such as audit or teaching, need more careful consideration. In addition to the standards discussed above, consideration should be given to whether the message of the recording could be achieved by any other means, for example, by using pictures of people who have mental capacity (and have given permission), by line drawing, verbal description or diagram; whether the patient could benefit from the recording being shown (for example, by the clinical team receiving other clinicians' suggestions on improving treatment); and whether other patients could benefit from the recording being shown (by educating other clinicians who treat similar patients).

Publications in clinical journals can be regarded as being in the public domain and therefore a more stringent consideration of the criteria discussed above is necessary and that there be greater evidence of the benefit of showing the recording. More difficult is the use of recordings for publicity purposes or for documentaries in newspapers or television. On the one hand there is the need to educate, while on the other hand the need exists to protect the individual. The starting point is that no recordings should be used for non-clinical purposes unless there are exceptional reasons for doing so. Where there is a proposed case for exception to this rule the following must be met:

- it must be clear that the message could not be achieved by using the picture of a person who had mental capacity and could give permission to the recording being used;
- it must be clear that the message is important enough to risk the confidentiality and privacy of the patient;
- there must be a very high level of probability that the patient would have agreed to have their picture shown.

## Conclusions and contemporary challenges presented by complex disabilities

Most of the more difficult ethical decisions in complex disabilities involve those people who lack mental capacity to make the decision required. One of the difficulties is that mental capacity is specific for the decision required. The main requirement is to act in the best interests of the individual, but that has considerable risks of imposing the values of able-bodied people. Sensitivity to the problems involved goes a long way towards providing the optimal ethical care for people with complex disabilities.

### References

Andrews, K., Murphy, L., Munday, R. and Littlewood, C. (1996) 'Misdiagnosis of the vegetative state: retrospective study in a rehabilitation unit', *British Medical Journal*, vol 313, pp 13–16.

Bach, J., Campagnolo, D. and Hoeman, S. (1991) 'Life satisfaction of individuals with Duchenne muscular dystrophy using long-term mechanical ventilatory support', *American Journal of Physical and Medical Rehabilitation*, vol 70, no 3, pp 129–35.

Beauchamp, T. and Childress, J. (2001) *Principles of biomedical ethics* (5th edn), New York, NY: Oxford University Press.

BMA (British Medical Association) (2001) *Withholding and withdrawing life-prolonging medical treatment: Guidance for decision making* (2nd edn), London: BMJ Books.

Childs, N., Mercer, W. and Childs, H. (1993) 'Accuracy of diagnosis of persistent vegetative state', *Neurology*, vol 43, pp 1465–67.

Cowley, C. (2004) 'The *Diane Pretty* case and the occasional impotence of justification in ethics', *Ethical Perspectives*, vol 11, no 4, pp 250–8.

DCA (Department for Constitutional Affairs) (2005) *The Mental Capacity Act (2005)*, London: The Stationery Office.

DH (Department of Health) (2004) *Mental Capacity Bill: Draft code of practice* (www.dca.gov.uk/menincap/mcbdraftcode.pdf).

Ebrahim, S. (2000) 'Do not resuscitate decisions: flogging dead horses or a dignified death?', *British Medical Journal*, vol 320, pp 1155–6.

GMC (General Medical Council) (2002) *Withholding and withdrawing life-prolonging treatments: Good practice in decision making*, London: GMC.

Hainsworth, D.S. (1998) 'Reflections on loss without death: the lived experience of acute care nurses caring for neurologically devastated patients', *Holistic Nursing Practitioner*, vol 13, no 1, pp 41–50.

Keown, J. (1997) 'Restoring moral and intellectual shape to the law after Bland', *Law Quarterly Review*, vol 113, pp 481–503.

Krumholz, H., Phillips, R., Hamel, M., Teno, J., Bellamy, P., Broste, S., Califf, R., Vidaillet, H., Davis, R., Muhlbaier, L., Connors, A. Jr., Lynn, J. and Goldman, L. (1998) 'Resuscitation preferences among patients with severe congestive heart failure: results from the SUPPORT project (Study to Understand Prognoses and Preferences for Outcomes and Risks of Treatment)', *Circulation*, vol 8, pp 648-55.

Levin, J., Wenger, N., Ouslander, J., Zellman, G., Schnelle, J., Buchanan, J., Hirsch, S. and Reuben, D. (1999) 'Life-sustaining treatment decisions for nursing home residents: who discusses, who decides and what is decided?', *Journal of the American Geriatric Society*, vol 47, pp 83-7.

Madl, C., Kramer, L., Yeganehfar, W.. Eisenhuber, E., Kranz, A., Ratheiser, K., Zauner, C., Schneider, B. and Grimm, G. (1996) 'Detection of nontraumatic comatose patients with no benefit of intensive care treatment by recording of sensory evoked potentials', *Archives of Neurology*, vol 53, no 6, pp 512-16.

Mariner, W. (1995) 'Rationing health care and the need for credible scarcity: why Americans can't say no', *American Journal of Public Health*, vol 85, no 10, pp 1439-45.

Menzel, P., Dolan, P., Richardson, J. and Olsen, J. (2002) 'The role of adaptation to disability and disease in health state valuation: a preliminary normative analysis', *Social Science and Medicine*, vol 55, no 12, pp 2149-58.

Mayo, D. and Gunderson, M. (2002) 'Vitalism revitalized ... vulnerable populations, prejudice, and physician-assisted death', *Hastings Centre Report*, vol 32, no 4, pp 14-21.

Mohr, M. and Kettler, D. (1997) 'Ethical conflicts in emergency medicine', *Anaesthetist*, vol 4, pp 275-81.

Morris, D. (2003) 'Assisted suicide under the European Convention on Human Rights: a critique', *European Human Rights Law Review*, vol 1, pp 65-91.

Pedain, A. (2003) 'The human rights dimension of the *Diane Pretty* case', *Cambridge Law Journal*, vol 62, no 1, pp 181-206.

Sayers, G., Schofield, I. and Aziz, M. (1997) 'An analysis of CPR decision-making by elderly patients', *Journal of Medical Ethics*, vol 23, pp 207-12.

Simonds, A. (2003) 'Ethics and decision making in end stage lung disease', *Thorax*, vol 58, no 3, pp 272-7.

Spittle, B. (1992) 'Paternalistic interventions with the gravely disabled', *Australian and New Zealand Journal of Psychiatry*, vol 26, no 1, pp 107-10.

Sullivan, M. (2003) 'The new subjective medicine: taking the patient's point of view on health care and health', *Social Science and Medicine*, vol 56, no 7, pp 1595-604.

Tresch, D., Farrol, H., Duthie, E., Goldstein, M. and Lane, P. (1991) 'Clinical characteristics of patients in the persistent vegetative state', *Archives of Internal Medicine*, vol 151, pp 930-2.

Uhlmann, R. and Pearlman, R. (1991) 'Perceived quality of life and preferences for life-sustaining treatment in older adults', *Archives of Internal Medicine*, vol 151, no 3, pp 495-7.

Weber, L. and Campbell, M. (1996) 'Medical futility and life-sustaining treatment decisions', *Journal of Neuroscience Nursing*, vol 28, no 1, pp 56-60.

White, S. and Baldwin, T. (2002) 'Miss B', *Anaesthesia*, vol 57, no 8, pp 818-19.

# SEVENTEEN

# Mental health: safe, sound and supportive?[1]

*Jon Glasby, Helen Lester and Emily McKie*[2]

## Summary

In 1998, the Department of Health (DH, 1998a) issued a White Paper on the future of mental health services. Entitled *Mental health: Safe, sound and supportive*, this document was the first in a series of official publications to outline fundamental reforms of health and social care for people with mental health problems (see, for example, DH, 1999a, 2001a). Subsequent measures included the introduction of national targets for adult mental health services, a new National Institute for Mental Health in England (NIMHE), additional investment and attempts to reform mental health legislation (the 1983 Mental Health Act; see DH, 1998b, 2001b, 2001c). Such activity in an area often seen as a 'Cinderella service' was almost unprecedented, yet was something of a mixed blessing. While mental health had long been campaigning for greater resources and recognition, this additional policy focus also highlighted a series of significant tensions. The White Paper suggested services were to be "safe, sound and supportive" (DH, 1998a), but largely failed to recognise that these factors may be different aspirations. In other words, can services, which are perceived as 'safe' by the public, media and politicians, also be perceived as 'supportive' by service users? More recently, the notion of patient choice has become key to NHS reforms (DH, 2003). In mental health, however, patient choice poses a key challenge, not least because the evolution of services has been influenced by the stigma of mental illness and coercive practices (Lester and Glasby, 2006). Against this background, this chapter examines the contested nature of mental health provision within the context of proposed legislative changes, exploring the key ethical dilemmas that are raised.

## Reform of the 1983 Mental Health Act

Frank Dobson's statement in the House of Commons on 29 July 1998 that "care in the community has failed" heralded a series of papers and consultation documents on the revision of the 1983 Mental Health Act. These papers included the *Report of the Expert Committee: Review of the Mental Health Act 1983* (DH, 1999b), chaired by Genevra Richardson and a Green Paper, *Reform of the Mental Health Act 1983: Proposals for consultation* (DH, 1999c). The Expert Committee argued that capacity, reciprocity, statutory rights to early advocacy and advanced statements needed to be recognised in future legislation. The Green Paper, however, largely ignored these recommendations and instead emphasised the need to manage risk in a paternalistic way, proposing new compulsory treatment orders (CTOs) for individuals posing a risk to self or others. The subsequent White Paper, *Reforming the Mental Health Act* (DH, 2001b, 2001c), attracted a great deal of attention, largely because of the overriding emphasis on public safety (Grounds, 2001).

The first Draft Mental Health Bill was published on 25 July 2002 (DH, 2002a, 2002b, 2002c). Although the Bill contained safeguards for certain patients treated informally, who are not capable of consenting, the Bill also proposed increased powers of compulsion. These proposals have created considerable concern for health and social care professionals, service users and wider society. Vociferous opposition has manifested, through the establishment of the Mental Health Alliance, an umbrella organisation of over 60 mental health groups.

The second (revised) Draft Mental Health Bill was published on 8 September 2004 (DH, 2004a). Despite modifications, critics still argue that services provided to an individual will be largely determined by the perceived risk these individuals pose to society rather than, as the Richardson report (DH, 1999b) proposed, their level of mental capacity (Mooney, 2004). Although the Bill has since been withdrawn, key concerns about these proposals include the following:

*The broad definition of mental disorder:* there is no single, universally accepted definition of mental illness. Unlike most physical illness, "knowledge is lacking on the aetiology of most disorders or on definitive treatment" (Mechanic, 1994, p 503). This situation has led to various definitions of mental illness, ranging from the purely social and purely biological to a combination of the two. The Draft Mental Health Bill (2004) defines mental disorder as "an impairment of or a disturbance in the functioning of the mind or brain resulting from any disability or disorder of the mind or brain" and in doing so adopts a bio-social model of mental disorder that significantly expands the definition from the 1983 Act. The result is that individuals with personality disorder or a diagnosis of alcohol/drug misuse may be included by the definition, potentially allowing far more people to be subject to compulsion than at present.

*The treatability clause:* this clause, enshrined in the 1959 Act and updated in the 1983 Act, implied that detention could be undertaken only if a commonly established treatment was available. The intention was to ensure that detention was for an individual's own benefit and not solely for the protection of society (Laurance, 2003, p 58). However, there is no clause in the revised Bill to state that treatment must be beneficial to the patient. Instead, medical treatment can be provided to protect a patient from suicide, serious self-harm, serious neglect of their health or safety, or of other people's safety. This outcome has particular implications for people diagnosed with dangerous and severe personality disorder living in the community, as the situation will allow non-offending people diagnosed with personality disorder to be detained indefinitely 'if clinically appropriate'. This position removes a dilemma from psychiatrists who have previously found themselves unable to treat a patient because it was not possible to say with complete confidence that the person's symptoms would improve. Indeed, 'untreatability' was the reason given for the non-detention of Michael Stone who went on to kill Lin Russell and her six-year-old daughter Megan in 1996. This single tragic act became a strong driving force for the reform of the 1983 Mental Health Act. However, by removing the treatability clause, powers of compulsion are significantly widened, to an arguably unjustifiable extent.

*Community treatment orders (CTOs):* CTOs mean patients can in practice be detained in the community. Patients required to attend for an injection or oral medication at a certain place and time, who fail to comply, might be removed to a clinical setting for drugs to be administered. This situation places real tensions on the notion of trust and therapeutic alliance within the doctor–patient relationship and user groups have warned that people may be driven away from services. Although the revised 2004 Mental Health Bill limits these extended powers so that only patients previously detained for inpatient care can be forcibly treated in the community and no time span is specified. CTOs also serve to demonstrate the well-recognised double standards in care between people with physical and mental health problems. Patients who are well enough to be in the community are generally well enough to make decisions for themselves even if the decision is not necessarily in the best interests of their health, a situation tolerated for someone with, for example, tuberculosis, but not with schizophrenia. These changes are also likely to increase the number of people subject to compulsion.

*Capacity:* impaired decision making is not a required condition for treatment to be enforced, which means that someone who has capacity and chooses not to take his or her medication could be compelled under the revised 2004 Draft Mental Health Bill. Once again, this situation serves to reinforce the double standards often applied to people with physical and mental illness.

*Workforce issues:* the extra appeals, tribunals and hearings that the new system may generate will require an estimated 1,000 additional staff, including an extra 130 psychiatrists (NHS Confederation, 2003) at a time when approximately 12% of consultant psychiatry posts in England and Wales are vacant.

## Ethical dilemmas

The reform of the 1983 Mental Health Act has raised a series of practical and ethical dilemmas for frontline practitioners in health and social services, service users and indeed for wider society. Some of these ethical dilemmas are outlined and explored below.

### Ethics of the 'mad' versus 'bad' debate

When someone commits a crime that the public finds particularly hard to understand, an immediate response is often to question if the person concerned is either 'mad' or 'bad'. Whereas many would see the need to punish the 'bad', people may often feel that someone with a mental health problem may not have been 'in their right mind' and hence not responsible for their action. As a result, such a person should receive treatment and care in the health service, rather than punishment in prison. In practice, such distinctions can be hard to make, particularly when the crime is horrific and difficult to comprehend. Examples include infamous figures such as Ian Brady, Myra Hindley and Ian Huntley. When accused of murdering the schoolgirls, Holly Wells and Jessica Chapman, Huntley was sectioned under the 1983 Mental Health

Act, assessed at a high security hospital, found not to have a mental health problem and, ultimately, convicted of murder. Clearly, this case was an extreme one, but one which does illustrate the profound importance of the mental health assessment, as someone with a mental health problem, assessed as not responsible for their actions, will 'escape' prison and be treated in a health rather than a penal setting. While viewed as part of the roles of particular mental health professionals, these matters are arguably more a philosophical question about the nature of 'evil' and the factors that can lead human beings to commit horrific crimes against each other. In extreme cases, such assessments can be about trying to surface the motives of a person who has committed a very serious crime and to unpick the thought processes of someone whose behaviour is virtually impossible to understand.

## Ethics of individual liberty versus public safety

Balancing the rights of individuals with mental illness and ensuring the welfare and safety of the wider public is a much-debated issue. From a moral perspective, all human beings are equal and therefore there should be equal concern for all people's well-being, equal respect for their autonomy and a desire to maximise these to the highest point compatible with basic equality (Campbell and Heginbotham, 1991, p 63). The current mental health system, however, permits a small percentage of people to be preventatively detained on the basis of posing a risk to themselves or others. Furthermore, the Draft Bill expands the numbers of people that might be preventatively detained by adopting a broader definition of mental illness, removing the treatability clause and extending powers of compulsion.

While seemingly reasonable to expect the government to pass laws that protect the rights of its citizens, these laws need to be balanced and proportionate to risk. Is it just to undermine individual autonomy in the interests of public safety (particularly given doubts about the accuracy of risk prediction)? If this view is justifiable, then at what point should action be taken? Or, from a different perspective, does the utilitarian ideal of the greatest good for the greatest number permit the deprivation of individual autonomy in an attempt to safeguard other people's fundamental rights, such as the right to life? These arenas present complex ethical dilemmas and involve important judgements about autonomy and beneficence. In the case of mental health services, however, a practical way forward may lie in a better understanding of risk and violence and the complexities of risk assessment.

There is a common misconception among many members of the public, often reinforced by the media, that mental health is necessarily linked to dangerousness and crime. Research suggests that two thirds of all British press and television coverage of mental health includes a link with violence, while around 40% of daily tabloid newspapers and nearly half of the Sunday tabloids contain derogatory references such as 'nutter' and 'loony' (ODPM, 2004, p 26). In the UK, media stereotypes have been fuelled by some very high profile and brutal murders. These human tragedies are terrible events, but are not representative cases. There is little evidence linking violence and mental illness (see, for example, Taylor and Gunn, 1999). Nonetheless, these cases have contributed to an enormous public outcry particularly about people with personality disorders, who have typically been portrayed as 'fiends' and 'perverts' (Markham, 2000, p 28).

Sayce (2000, p 226) summarises some key facts that should be borne in mind when discussing mental health and crime:

- most crime is committed by people without mental health problems;
- where people with mental health problems commit crimes, the reason is often the same as for everyone else (poverty, drink and drugs, family/relationship frustrations);
- for people with mental health problems to attack someone unknown to themselves is extremely rare;
- people with mental health problems are more often victims than perpetrators of crime;
- people with mental health problems can usually be held responsible for their crimes.

Furthermore, in their evidence submitted to the Joint Committee on the Draft Mental Health Bill, the Royal College of Psychiatrists (2003) stated that for each citizen killed by a person with mental ill health, 10 are killed by corporate manslaughter, 20 by people who are not mentally ill, 25 by passive smoking and 125 by NHS hospital-acquired infection.

To predict risk accurately is also extremely difficult, if not impossible. As Peck (quoted in Chamberlain, 1998, p 2) observes:

> The assessment of risk and dangerousness is an art not a science and a difficult art which requires practitioners to balance past and present behaviour with predictions of interventions and the civil liberties of the patient.

Using statistics from the National Confidential Inquiry, Laurance (2003, pp 67-9) has calculated that implementing the 2004 Mental Health Bill would result in 32 suicides and 3 homicides per year being prevented. At the same time, Moller (2002) notes that the Bill could potentially result in the preventative detention of 5,000 innocent people to prevent one homicide (Moller, 2002), with 100 people detained to prevent one suicide. As such, the Bill would appear to result in substantial suffering for some people in order to provide benefits to a much smaller number of others. Given the fundamental principles outlined above, this outcome is morally unacceptable: "equality and fairness should take precedence over maximisation of utility, even though we may not get as much total well-being in society as a whole" (Campbell and Heginbotham, 1991, p 90).

Undoubtedly there is a point where people need protecting from harm; failure to do so would violate the principle of equal concern and respect (Campbell and Heginbotham, 1991, p 2). However, if autonomy is seen as of primary importance with paternalism an important secondary guide, the revised Draft Bill fails to reflect these principles.

## Ethics of care versus control

In many ways, the title of *Safe, sound and supportive* (DH, 1998a) summarises a long-standing tension in health and social care between services that care for people in distress and services that seek to control individual behaviour. For example, social workers concerned about the welfare of a newborn baby can initiate child protection proceedings that can lead to the child being taken into the care of the local authority; a person with a profound learning disability can be placed under guardianship or can have their affairs handled via powers of attorney; a frail older person living in conditions hazardous to health can, in a limited number of settings, be removed from their own home under the 1948 National Assistance Act; and people with mental health problems can be 'sectioned' (that is, compulsorily admitted to hospital, assessed and treated, potentially against their will). In some situations, these steps may be necessary to protect individuals; in other cases these measures may be experienced as unnecessary interference and an invasion of personal liberty.

Critics of the revised Draft Bill argue that the proposed legislation will force health professionals to operate far more as public protectors than therapists (Eastman, 1999), particularly with the threshold for public safety increased so that a patient with mental illness can be compelled 'for the protection of other persons', which does not necessarily mean there is a significant risk to others. The Medical Defence Union has expressed concern that, in applying the Draft Bill, doctors might contravene their own code of ethics, which requires all interventions to be in the best interests of the patient.

## Patient choice agenda in mental health

As outlined above, the Draft Mental Health Bill raises significant ethical issues with regard to autonomy, beneficence and individual liberty. At the same time, there is also a danger that current proposals for reform deny mental health service users access to the same principles and quality of care as other NHS patients. Nowhere is this more clearly illustrated than in the case of patient choice.

Under New Labour, the patient choice agenda was formalised in policy terms through *The NHS Plan* (DH, 2000), which emphasised the government's commitment to creating a patient-centred NHS with users' needs central to service design and delivery:

> Patients are the most important people in the health service. It doesn't always appear that way. Too many patients feel talked at, rather than listened to. This has to change. NHS care has to be shaped around the convenience and concerns of patients. To bring this about, patients must have more say in their own treatment and more influence over the way the NHS works. (DH, 2000, p 88)

More recently, Dr John Reid, the former Secretary of State for Health, stated "Trust me, I'm a patient, should be the guiding principle of the new agenda" and promised that the choice agenda would effectively turn the traditional doctor-centred health service on its head (Reid, 2003). In practical terms, current goals in the choice agenda include the ability of all patients to be able to choose between four or five different providers for elective care by December 2005 (DH, 2004b) and to opt to be seen at another hospital if on a waiting list for elective surgery for longer than six months.

This patient choice agenda raises a number of issues and creates particular tensions for people with mental health problems since choice appears to vary according to who is choosing, what choices are available and the supporting policy infrastructure. The government has stated that "the choice agenda applies as much to mental health services as anywhere else" (Winterton, 2004), although the opportunity to 'choose and book' appointments does not currently apply to mental health (DH, 2004b) and there is no alternative choice for patients who have waited more than six months for treatment (usually for psychological therapies).

Although there are some elements of patient choice within the revised Draft Bill, such as access to an independent advocacy service to help patients assert their rights, choice of nominated representative (who until now has always been the closest relative) and the right to refuse electroconvulsive therapy if the person is felt to retain their mental capacity, the majority of proposed changes fail to reflect the broader principles underpinning the patient choice agenda.

In 2003-04, the 1983 Mental Health Act was used on 45,700 occasions (DH, 2005). This figure is relatively small when compared with the overall number of people with serious mental illness at any one time (630,000), but has a disproportionate effect on how clinicians and society view people with mental illness and indeed how patients view services (Perkins and Repper, 1998). The proposed changes may serve to reinforce further a culture of compulsion rather than patient choice, with coercion extended beyond the inpatient setting to the community and to a greater number of people because of the broader definition of mental disorder. The prevalent blame culture within medicine also means that psychiatrists are increasingly unlikely to take any sort of risk with their reputation or decision making even if that means further reducing patients' choice by using a CTO (Community Treatment Order).

## Conclusions and contemporary challenges for mental health

This chapter has argued that proposed changes to the 1983 Mental Health Act are focused on risk and public safety rather than on the health and welfare of those people whose decision making is impaired by reason of their mental disorder. The 2004 Draft Mental Health Bill is also out of step with other current relevant government policy initiatives in this area, particularly the choice agenda, which risks disadvantaging people with mental health problems relative to other patient groups.

In addition, the currently proposed legislation risks creating a system where voluntary patients fear using the system and where the services available to these patients are limited because resources are focused on the increasing number of people under compulsion. A better starting point for risk reduction is to encourage patients to feel able to seek help early, to talk about their fears and problems and then engage with services that are accessible, effective, appropriate and responsive. This approach would not only be better for individual service users, but may also be a more effective form of protection for the wider public.

Whatever happens to current mental health legislation, this chapter has argued that future services will need to address a series of underlying ethical issues and contemporary challenges:

- Why do some people commit horrific crimes and how can we understand their motivations and thought processes?
- How can we best balance individual liberty and autonomy with public safety and the right to life?
- In whose interest should services be provided and at what stage does the state have a moral right and duty to impose services on individuals, either for their own 'good' or for the safety of others?

Unfortunately, current proposals seem to be overlooking some of these fundamental issues altogether. Furthermore, the mental health system seems as far away as ever from finding genuine and ethically acceptable answers to these questions.

## Note

[1] This chapter draws in part on a summary of the literature on forensic mental health services published in H. Lester and J. Glasby (2006) *Mental health policy and practice*, Basingstoke: Palgrave.

[2] The views expressed in this chapter are entirely personal and are not necessarily those of the organisations for which Emily McKie works.

## References

Campbell, T. and Heginbotham, C. (1991) *Mental illness: Prejudice, discrimination and the law*, Aldershot: Dartmouth Publishing Company Ltd.

Chamberlain, L. (1998) 'Murdered worker's family win apology from Kingston', *Community Care*, 9–15 July, p 2.

DH (Department of Health) (1998a) *Modernising mental health services: Safe, sound and supportive*, London: DH.

DH (1998b) 'Frank Dobson outlines a third way for mental health', Press Release 98/311, London: DH.

DH (1999a) *National service framework for mental health: Modern standards and service models*, London: DH.

DH (1999b) *Report of the Expert Committee: Review of the Mental Health Act 1983* (the Richardson Report), London: DH.

DH (1999c) *Reform of the Mental Health Act 1983: Proposals for consultation*, London: The Stationery Office.

DH (2000) *The NHS Plan: A plan for investment, a plan for reform*, London: DH.

DH (2001a) *Safety first: Five-year report of the National Confidential Inquiry into suicide and homicide by people with mental illness*, London: DH.

DH (2001b) *Reforming the Mental Health Act – Part I: The new legal framework*, London: DH.

DH (2001c) *Reforming the Mental Health Act – Part II: High risk patients*, London: DH.

DH (2002a) *Draft Mental Health Bill*, Cm 5538-I, London: The Stationery Office.

DH (2002b) *Draft Mental Health Bill, Explanatory Notes*, Cm 5538-II, London: The Stationery Office.

DH (2002c) *Mental Health Bill Consultation Document*, Cm 5538-III, London: The Stationery Office.

DH (2003) *Building on the best: Choice, responsiveness and equity in the NHS*, London: The Stationery Office.

DH (2004a) *Draft Mental Health Bill*, Cm 6305-1, London: DH.

DH (2004b) *Choose and book: Patient's choice of hospital and booked appointment*, London: DH.

DH (2005) *Detentions under the Mental Health Act 1983, in admission and subsequent to admission in NHS facilities (including high security psychiatric hospitals) England 1987-88 and 2003-4*, London: DH.

Eastman, N. (1999) 'Public health psychiatry or crime prevention?', *British Medical Journal*, vol 318, pp 549-51.

Grounds, A. (2001) 'Reforming the Mental Health Act', *British Journal of Psychiatry*, vol 178, pp 387-9.

Laurance, J. (2003) *Pure madness: How fear drives the mental health system*, London: Routledge.

Lester, H. and Glasby, J. (2006) *Mental health: Policy and practice*, Basingstoke: Palgrave.

Markham, G. (2000) 'Policy and service development trends: forensic mental health and social care services', *Tizard Learning Disability Review*, vol 5, no 2, pp 26-31.

Mechanic, D. (1994) 'Establishing mental health priorities', *The Milbank Quarterly*, vol 72, no 3, pp 501-14.

Moller, C. (2002) 'Comment: mad, bad and dangerous law', *The Guardian*, 27 June.

Mooney, H. (2004) 'Mental health changes slammed', *Health Service Journal*, 9 September, p 5.

NHS Confederation (2003) *The Draft Mental Health Bill: An assessment of the implications for mental health service organisations*, London: NHS Confederation.

ODPM (Office of the Deputy Prime Minister) (2004) *Mental health and social exclusion*, Social Exclusion Unit Report, London: ODPM.

Perkins, R. and Repper, J. (1998) *Dilemmas in community mental health practice: Choice or control*, Abingdon: Radcliffe Medical Press.

Reid, J. (2003) Choice speech to New Health Network, 16 July, London: DH.

Royal College of Psychiatrists (2003) *Reform of mental health legislation* (available at www.rcpsych.ac.uk/press/parliament/MHBill.htm, accessed 21/06/2005).

Sayce, L. (2000) *From psychiatric patient to citizen: Overcoming discrimination and social exclusion*, Basingstoke: Palgrave.

Taylor, P. and Gunn, J. (1999) 'Homicides by people with mental illness: myth and reality', *British Journal of Psychiatry*, vol 174, pp 9-14.

Winterton, R. (2004) Speech to Sainsbury Centre for Mental Health and Warwick Medical School, 13 July.

# EIGHTEEN

# Ethics and older people

*Anthea Tinker*

## Summary

There are two main areas where ethical issues arise for older people in health and social care. The first relates to services and the second to research. This chapter will start with general issues, such as general and demographic factors, in order to examine the ethical case for and against treating older people differently from other age groups. Are there groups, such as those with dementia, who should receive different attention? On services, ethical issues such as those relating to age discrimination and changing views on autonomy will be examined. On research, ethical procedures (including consent, confidentiality and the role of older people on ethics committees) will be considered in the context of both formal and informal arrangements.

## Defining older people

There is no agreement about the definition of older people. Some take pensionable age while others use chronological age such as all people over the age of 65 or 70. Ethically it could be argued that taking a chronological age is the 'fairest' because of being less likely to be challenged than something more ill defined. Of interest is a new concept to emerge which is argued as 'fairer' and that is biological or 'real' age. The proponents argue that physical and mental health can be measured and that, while a person may be 60 chronologically, these individuals are some other age physically and mentally. Others argue that image defines an older person. Those who look and act 'old' are old. It is also argued that the definition changes with different periods of time and with varied cultures. For example, in some cultures people would define themselves as 'old' at a comparatively early age either because of shorter lifespans or because of the veneration associated with old age.

The importance of definitions arises because of a perceived 'fairness' or 'justice' over the provision of services and for how older people are treated. Legal and moral rights flow from the definitions. Some of the definitions of ethics, that is, 'science of morals' and 'moral principles or codes', are arguably not set in tablets of stone but subject to interpretation according to a culture and a period of time. For older people there are examples of cultural differences that can profoundly affect both services and research. At one extreme are attitudes to death and at the other views about parts of the body such as hair and nail clippings.

## Demographic challenge of an ageing population

The relative size of a group will impinge on ethical issues because of the potential threat (or challenge) for that group to exercise power. There are three practical facts that will impact on the provision of services and the subsequent potential ethical dilemmas. These facts are:

- the increased numbers of older people;
- the increased proportion of older people;
- the decline of support ratios.

Table 18.1 shows both the actual and projected *numbers* of older people; that includes the projected rise in numbers of both 'younger' old people and those who are 'older'.

Table 18.2 shows both the actual and projected *proportions* of older people and the projected rise in the proportion of older people.

**Table 18.1:** Actual and projected numbers of older people in the UK (millions)

|                  | 2002 | 2026 |
|------------------|------|------|
| Aged 60-74       | 7.9  | 11.0 |
| Aged 75 and over | 4.5  | 7.1  |

*Source:* Government Actuary's Department (2002, p 8)

**Table 18.2:** Actual and projected proportions of older people in the UK (percentages)

|                  | 2002 | 2026 |
|------------------|------|------|
| Aged 60-74       | 13.3 | 17.2 |
| Aged 75 and over | 7.5  | 11.1 |

*Source:* Government Actuary's Department (2002, p 8)

**Table 18.3:** Actual and projected people of pensionable age* per 1,000 people of working age

|  | 2002 | 2026 |
| --- | --- | --- |
|  | 291 | 331 |

*Note:* * Pension age population is based on state retirement age for the given year. Between 2010 and 2020 state retirement age will change from 65 years for men and 60 years for women to 65 years for both sexes.

*Source:* Government Actuary's Department (2004, p A 3)

Table 18.3 shows the actual and projected numbers of *dependants* for people of pensionable age per 1,000 people of working age. This shows that those of pensionable age will increase as a proportion of those of working age.

What all these figures show are two conflicting possible ethical dilemmas. First, the obvious growing voting power of older people, but, second, their possible dependence on a shrinking proportion of people of working age. Although there is little evidence in the UK that the growing proportion of older people are seeking to exercise a self-interested power, this development could be an ethical dilemma. However, there is some evidence that the reverse is true with some older people expressing more concern about education and issues to do with younger age groups than their own self-interest. The exception is the widespread concern by older people about their pensions. If pensions are to be provided out of public money, that is, the taxpayers', then the latter are entitled to argue that their generation have not had many of the benefits that their parents and grandparents received such as help with mortgage repayments and free university education.

## Are older people a special group and, if so, why?

If there is no agreed definition of older people, why should this group be treated differently? For practical purposes such as eligibility for a pension or bus pass it is simpler to state an age rather than some other complicated method. Much of the argument for treating older people as a special group rests on the premise that this age group are more likely to have physical and mental disabilities. There is some evidence that this is the case *on average* (see Table 18.4).

The greater risk of dementia in old age is another factor. While 5% of people over the age of 65 have dementia, the rate for those aged 85 and over is 20%.

Both greater mental and physical ill health are indicators of the greater likelihood of the need for services. However, many older people

**Table 18.4:** Some indicators of age and disability (all self-reported) (2001)

| Aged | 45-64 | 65-74 | 75+ |
|---|---|---|---|
| % with long-standing illness | 43 | 57 | 63 |
| Acute sickness – average number of restricted activity days per person | 41 | 50 | 75 |
| Hospital inpatient in 12 months before interview (%) | 8 | 11 | 17 |

*Source:* Office for National Statistics (2002, pp 89, 91, 112)

are in good health and more able to cope than those who are younger but more disabled, which presents an argument for the provision of services based on physical and mental ability.

The arguments for treating older people as a special group in the provision of services can be summarised as:

- most will have ceased work;
- there is a moral and expected obligation, for example, for the provision of a pension;
- an intergenerational contract (whether formally stated or not) has led to the expectation of some services based on what has happened in the past;
- some groups, such as those with dementia, will have special needs;
- these groups may be vulnerable because of their physical or mental disability or their living circumstances.

However, there are also arguments on the other side which are:

- many older people are in good health and may be in better health than some younger people;
- many older people will want to be in paid employment and will be capable of undertaking this;
- it is discriminatory to treat older people differently;
- society has changed and there is no longer an ethical or moral obligation for younger generations to support older ones.

## Ethical issues in the provision of health and social care

Justice (or fairness) is held to be one of the main principles of ethics (see Thiroux, 1980). Equity is currently a more common description of fairness. The main ethical issue in the provision of health and social care (apart from those to do with end of life issues, which are considered in Chapter Nineteen) is equity of treatment/care. Is treatment and care to be given on the basis of need? Are there circumstances in which the age of a person should be taken into account and, if so, what are the circumstances? Are older people advantaged or disadvantaged and, if so, what is the basis for this? In some cases age per se is used as the criteria for eligibility: for example for flu and pneumonia jabs or bus passes. In the first case, others are included such as those with particular health problems. But services such as the provision of bus passes are given on a blanket basis regarding age alone. The extra fuel allowance and free television licence are other examples of services provided purely on the basis of age but without a means test. One argument is that older people have 'earned' these free services based on age, but ethically another argument is that others are more in need. In these cases, older people are at an advantage and the subject of positive discrimination.

In addition older people are also more likely to receive a higher proportion of health and social services than their proportion in the population would 'justify'. For example, people over the age of 65 represent 16% of the population yet received 46% of local authority social services expenditure in 2000/01 (ONS, 2002, p 149).

The other side of the coin is where older people are the subject of age discrimination which is clearly an ethical issue. Plenty of evidence of age discrimination exists in health and social care, as well as considerable evidence of age discrimination in employment, but this is beyond the scope of this chapter.

A definition of age discrimination is not easy. The King's Fund auditing study mentioned some of the different kinds including direct and indirect, ageist attitudes and the way that the issues are compounded by factors such as 'race', disability and gender (Levenson, 2003).

Evidence about discrimination in health and social care began to mount in the early 1990s with the ground-breaking book *Age: The unrecognised discrimination*, edited by the late Evelyn McEwen (McEwen, 1990). Although the publication was subtitled *Views to provoke a debate*, the authors provided evidence but, more importantly, pointed to the roots of the problem as being ageism. In a perceptive chapter 'The foundation of age discrimination', Steve Scrutton (1990) describes a depressing and widely held view of old age as the foundation on which judgements are made about an individual's worth, but explained the social creation of ageism as being based on the loss of physical strength and the declining value placed on acquired knowledge and experience. In the same book Melanie Henwood argued that "There is no doubt that the chronic and long term needs of older people receive inadequate attention at the present... Ethical debates about the quality of life and the limits of medical intervention are certain to become more pressing as frontiers are rolled back on what is technically possible" (Henwood, 1990, p 56).

This publication was followed up by research with the telling title *Turning your back on us: Older people and the NHS* (National Health Service) (Gilchrist, 1999), which provided accounts of discrimination. Evidence continued to mount about age discrimination in health and social care in the 1990s. There are now clear government guidelines to the contrary. The *National Service Framework* (NSF) *for older people* was stated by the Minister of Health in his Foreword to be a 10-year programme "to ensure fair, high quality, integrated health and social care services for older people" (DH, 2001a, p 1), which was to be done by laying down eight standards. The first was 'rooting out age discrimination'. The Department of Health stated that "NHS services will be provided, regardless of age, on the basis of clinical need alone. Social care services will not use age in their eligibility criteria or policies, to restrict access to available services" (DH, 2001a, p 16).

This statement was followed by more specific advice in some areas, for example, in *Medicines and older people: Implementing medicine-related aspects of the national service framework* (DH, 2001b). The interim report on age discrimination by the Department of Health in April 2002 found a raised awareness of the topic but still considerable variation in practice. A subsequent follow-up showed that only a small number of NHS bodies still had written policies that discriminated against older people. There were some examples of good practice but action was now needed "to root out unwritten, implicit age discrimination" (DH, 2003, p 11).

Research undertaken by the King's Fund in late 2001 on senior managers working in health and social services in England found that:

- three out of four senior managers believed that age discrimination existed in some form or other in services in their local areas;
- many believed that ageism was endemic;
- some gave examples of discrimination that they felt were justified or favoured older people;
- only around a quarter of respondents felt that there was little or no age discrimination within local services (Roberts et al, 2002, Executive Summary).

The King's Fund concluded that the NSF, with its emphasis on written policies, will not challenge ageist organisational cultures and attitudes in the short term at least and further strategies are required.

The Department of Health followed up the NSF with an audit of NHS organisations in 2002 (DH, 2002). The Department of Health claimed that the audit has:

- raised awareness of age discrimination as an important issue;
- gained considerable support within the NHS and social care areas;
- shown that a very small number of policies explicitly discriminate on the basis of age;
- identified a lack of a common definition or wide understanding of age discrimination and this impedes actions to end such discrimination;
- revealed that undertaking an audit is complex and time consuming.

The main voluntary bodies with a concern about older people, Age Concern and Help the Aged, have been at the forefront of campaigns to stop age discrimination and have undertaken research on this topic. In 2002 Help the Aged gave the following examples of age discrimination from health care (Help the Aged, 2002):

- explicit – examples of where age cut-offs deny older people access to services, for example, the upper age limit for routine breast screening, to coronary care units and cardiac rehabilitation units;
- subtler forms – evidence of negative attitudes by staff to older people, the misdiagnosis or neglect of depression and other forms of mental illness;
- indirect – the low priority to chronic health conditions, the lack of an alternative to the NHS provided by private health insurance.

This evidence was reinforced by later research, which again highlighted difficulties in accessing medical care, being denied medical treatment, being placed in hospital wards offering poor, or non-specialist care and disbelief when describing symptoms or being misdiagnosed (Help the Aged, 2004).

In a review of the evidence on discrimination on social care, Melanie Henwood (2002, p 72) maintains that:

- Despite the welcome stance of the NSF in putting age discrimination at the top of its agenda it is apparent that in many ways discrimination is institutionalised.

- Areas of both direct and indirect discrimination are evident in social care services from cost ceilings that are habitually set at a lower level for the support of older people, to charging policies that have a disproportionate impact on older people and the underdevelopments of 'low level' services that have a greater potential in sustaining the independence of older people.

Older people have also identified age discrimination by social care workers, having their needs ignored and being recipients of poor standards of care (Help the Aged, 2004).

A recent overt example of discrimination is the guidance issued by the National Institute for Clinical Excellence (NICE), which provides guidance on health issues. In a controversial consultation paper in May 2005, NICE (2005) in a press release first recommended that:

- "Health should not be valued more highly in some age groups rather than others."
- "Individuals' social roles, at different ages, should not influence considerations of cost effectiveness."

But the third criterion was:

- "Where age is an indicator of benefit or risk, age discrimination may be appropriate" (NICE, 2005).

Not for the first time have people argued that age is an appropriate criterion for choosing which people could benefit from health care. For example, a distinguished economist, discussing high-tech interventions, said that "This vain pursuit of immortality is dangerous for elderly people: taken to its logical conclusion it implies that no one should be allowed to die until everything possible has been done. That means not simply that we shall all die in hospital but that we shall die in intensive care" (Williams, 1997, p 820). The chair of NICE has subsequently made this general point: "The NHS, like every other healthcare system in the world, has finite resources. The ethical issue is how – not whether – these resources should be fairly distributed. Neither rigid adherence to utilitarianism nor unqualified egalitarianism meet the needs of the NHS and the people it serves" (Rawlins, 2005, p 22).

Research shows that the reasons for age discrimination are:

- lack of resources
- widespread ageism in society
- the legacy of historical ageism in the welfare state (Roberts et al, 2002, p 24).

Running through the debate about discrimination in services, a salutary reminder comes from an older person that at the heart of the ethical dilemma is attitudes. Joan Simey (2002, pp 2–3) wrote:

> It is the denial of our need to belong, to have the security of a recognised place in society, however insignificant, that is so demeaning, so demoralising.... We have to believe that we are of some worth, have some right to a place in the life of the community. That is our human heritage. Deny us that and both we and the community to which we belong must surely perish.

The move to consumerism and the involvement of people in the running of services is an interesting ethical one. How easily can a representative older person be obtained to serve on a committee? On how many committees is there the statutory older person who becomes almost a professional 'older person'? On the other hand, some voluntary posts are available where to have the views of the whole community is desirable, such as magistrates, but where there is an upper age limit.

## Ethical issues in research on older people

As with services, the key question in research is whether older people should be treated differently from other age groups. There may be good reasons why older people should be included as a vulnerable group. If older people are physically frail, have dementia or are in an institution, there may be reasons for considering their position specially. In general, however, older people should have the same rights and responsibilities as people of other ages. Mary Gilhooly (2002, p 211) puts the case:

> In one sense there is nothing special about researching later life, or research with older people. Most older people live independent lives, are self-determining and are competent to decide whether or not to take part in research. They should be treated in the same way that one would treat any other adult asked to take part in research and the

ethical issues that arise are no different than they are when conducting research with younger adults.

However Gilhooly (2002) also gave some examples where there may be reasons for different treatment or where particular issues are raised.

Ethical issues may arise over the choice of sample. One of the most serious ethical issues is the exclusion of older people from clinical trials. This situation can affect prescribing. For example "If the evidence base for prescribing is so poor that the physician may be torn between prescribing on the basis of an extrapolation from the results of trials in younger patients, or not prescribing with the risk of being characterised as ageist" (Crome and Pollock, 2005, p 1). But there are other issues. For example, older people are often easier to study when they are not difficult to find, such as in sheltered housing or a care home. For those who are in some kind of protected environment, such as a care home, there may be suspicion, that, however the researchers claim the information given to be confidential, the information will get back to those who run the establishment. There may also be covert pressure to take part and possibly to give acceptable answers. On the other hand, older people may be 'protected' by a gatekeeper such as a warden who is reluctant to allow this group to be involved.

Also a further argument is that this generation of older people are more compliant than younger ones and are more likely to consent to taking part in research. To choose a sample on this basis again poses ethical dilemmas.

The exclusion of certain groups from research is also an ethical matter. Boneham (2002, p 208) argues that the cultural context for ageing has not been sufficiently taken into account. Where minority older people are not in contact with existing service providers, there may be challenges for a researcher in obtaining a representative sample and in gaining credibility for his or her research. Minority communities have suffered in the past from having their needs dismissed through ignorance or apathy and not being involved in the design of research about their own members.

The issues of consent, confidentiality and autonomy must also be considered. 'Informed consent' is needed so that participants can make an autonomous decision. Consent to taking part in the research, whether involving physical tests such as taking blood, or answering questionnaires, is at the heart of good ethical practice. Making sure that the participant understands what the research is about, what the procedures are, what will happen to the data and so on are important for people of every age. The Department of Health in *12 key points on consent: The law in England* (DH, 2001c) gives general guidelines for health professionals. Paragraph 2 states that:

> Adults are always assumed to be competent unless demonstrated otherwise. If you have any doubts about their competence, the question to ask is: 'Can this patient understand and weigh up the information needed to make this decision?'. Unexpected decisions do not prove that the patient is incompetent, but may indicate a need for further information or explanation.

While this view applies to the patient–health professional situation, other guidance from the Department of Health in *Seeking consent, working with older people* states: "The same principles apply to seeking consent for research as for consent to treatment. Patients who have the capacity to give or withhold consent to research will decide for themselves whether or not they wish to participate" (DH, 2001d, p 13). Most of the special measures that may be needed for older people, such as larger print information sheets, would also be needed for people with sight problems. At older ages this problem is likely to be more prevalent.

Unjustifiable pressure must not occur, that is, when someone in authority urges a course of action to the participant (Belmont Report, 1978). Research on sensitive subjects, such as domestic violence, sexual orientation and family relationships, needs care for people of all ages. However, for older people elder abuse, coming out as a gay older person or failing relationships within the family may be particularly sensitive to a generation less used to talking about such matters. Memory tests such as the mini mental test may cause anxiety (see Tinker, 1997).

A further matter is the role of older people on research committees. There is no age limit on members of local research ethics committees. There is no evidence about an upper age limit for university research ethics committees but, given their great variety, there is unlikely to be a consensus on the matter of an age limit (Tinker and Coomber, 2004).

## Conclusions and contemporary challenges presented by ethics and older people

Care should be taken not to assume that older people are different from those of other ages. Examples have been given where older people may have different characteristics and therefore treated differently, but, in most cases, this outcome is for other reasons. If older people are vulnerable because of physical or mental disability this should be the criteria and not age. Many of the ethical issues to do with older people relate to an ageing population. The change in the relative balance numerically between old and young highlights issues of power and whether this is related to size. Ethically it is argued that older people should be treated the same as any age group, for example, not be discriminated against, have the same rights and responsibilities and be included in research. The reality, as this chapter has shown, is far from this situation. However, the growing proportion of older people, and their important contribution to society, will make this position harder to defend.

### Ethical disclosure

The author undertakes research with and on older people. She is also a participant in a longitudinal study and therefore has personal experience of being an older person in a research project.

### References

Belmont Report (1978) *Ethical principles and guidelines for the protection of human subjects of research*, Washington DC: US Department of Health, Education and Welfare.

Boneham, M. (2002) 'Researching ageing in different cultures', in A. Jamieson and C. Victor, *Researching ageing and later life*, London: Open University Press, pp 198-210.

Crome, P. and Pollock, K. (2005) 'Age discrimination in prescribing: accounting for concordance', *Reviews in Clinical Gerontology*, vol 14, no 1, pp 1-4.

DH (Department of Health) (2001a) *National service framework for older people*, London: DH.

DH (2001b) *Medicines and older people: Implementing medicine-related aspects of the national service framework*, London: DH.

DH (2001c) *12 key points on consent: The law in England* (www.doh.gov.uk/consent/twelvekeypoints.htm).

DH (2001d) *Seeking consent: Working with older people*, London: DH.

DH (2002) *National service framework for older people: Interim report on age discrimination* (contact A.J.Fenyo@ukc.ac.uk).

DH (2003) *National service framework for older people: A report of progress and future challenges*, London: DH.

Gilchrist, C. (1999) *Turning your back on us: Older people and the NHS*, London: Age Concern.

Gilhooly, M. (2002) 'Ethical issues in researching later life', in A. Jamieson and C.Victor, *Researching ageing and later life*, London: Open University Press, pp 211-25.

GAD (Government Actuary's Department) (2002) *Population projections 2000-2070*, London: GAD.

GAD (2004) *National Population Projections 2002 – based*, London: The Stationery Office.

Help the Aged (2002) *Age discrimination in public policy: A review of the evidence*, London: Help the Aged.

Help the Aged (2004) *Everyday age discrimination: The experience of older people*, London: Help the Aged.

Henwood, M. (1990) 'No sense of urgency: age discrimination in health care', in E. McEwen, *Age: The unrecognised discrimination: Views to provoke a debate*, London: Age Concern, pp 43-57.

Henwood, M. (2002) 'Age discrimination in health care', in Help the Aged, *Age discrimination in public policy: A review of the evidence*, London: Help the Aged, pp 71-88.

Levenson, R. (2003) *Auditing age discrimination*, London: King's Fund.

McEwen, E. (1990) *Age: The unrecognised discrimination: Views to provoke a debate*, London: Age Concern.

NICE (National Institute for Clinical Excellence) (2005) 'NICE consultation on social value judgements', Press release, London: NICE.

ONS (Office for National Statistics) (2002) *Living in Britain: Results from the 2001 General Household Survey*, London: The Stationery Office.

Rawlins, M. (2005) Letter to *The Times*, 8 October, p 22.

Roberts, E., Robinson, J. and Seymour, L. (2002) *Old habits die hard*, London: King's Fund.

Scrutton, S. (1990) 'The foundations of age discrimination', in E. McEwen, *Age: The unrecognised discrimination: Views to provoke a debate*, London: Age Concern, pp 12-27.

Simey, M. (2002) 'Foreword', in Help the Aged, *Age discrimination in public policy: A review of the evidence*, London: Help the Aged, pp 1-4.

Thiroux, J. (1980) *Ethics: Theory and practice*, California: Glencoe Publishing Company Inc.

Tinker, A. (1997) 'The other side of the fence', *British Medical Journal*, vol 315, no 7119, pp 1385-6.

Tinker, A. and Coomber, V. (2004) *University research ethics committees: Their role, remit and conduct*, London: The Nuffield Foundation.

Williams, A. (1997) 'Rationing health care by age: the case for', *British Medical Journal*, vol 314, pp 820-2.

# NINETEEN

# Ethics and euthanasia

*Clive Seale*

## Summary

Public support for laws that allow medical practitioners to end life by active measures has risen in recent years, but the medical profession in the UK has been reluctant to endorse this development. The obvious benefits to a few people who experience extremes of suffering towards the end of life need to be balanced against the interests of those who might feel pressurised to opt for death in a society where euthanasia becomes an acceptable and well-known solution to the problems of old age. Additionally, the effect on practitioners (usually doctors) who are called on to administer lethal treatments requires consideration. This chapter reports surveys of the relatives and friends of people who have died, as well as surveys of medical practitioners, to provide empirical evidence that deepens understanding of how moral and ethical dilemmas play themselves out in practice.

## Introduction

End of life decision making requires consideration of numerous potential harms and benefits that may arise from particular decisions. Some of these consequences may be immediate, obvious and personal. For example, there are obvious benefits in relieving an individual's suffering and in avoiding inappropriate life-sustaining therapies. Other harms and benefits are less obvious and often unintended. For example, potential harm may be done to efforts to establish good palliative care services if the option of legal euthanasia is available. There may be harms involved in allowing a system that places pressure on vulnerable people to opt for euthanasia. On the other hand it may be argued that in a system that permits medical actions to end life there are beneficial effects of open disclosure that allows scrutiny of these actions.

For the general public of media–saturated countries like the UK, the more obvious consequences are more easily appreciated. Mass media therefore often focus on these outcomes, providing a diet of personalised stories of end of life care that generally demonstrate the benefits of relieving individual suffering through acts of euthanasia (McInerney, 2000; Hausmann, 2004). Coupled with a general decline in religious attachment and the rise in rationalist and consumerist ideologies, the overall effect, in recent years, has been to raise levels of public support for legal measures that allow medical practitioners to end life by active measures (Seale, 1997). It is harder and apparently less appealing to most consumers of mass media to explain the less obvious and often harmful consequences of such policies, or to describe the negative impact that such actions may have on those given the task of carrying them out.

Capacities to make decisions and follow them through with actions are frequently constrained, by physical or mental capacity for example, or by legal and professional proscriptions. Cultural and ideological factors, such as the degree of attachment to religious as against rationalist belief systems, or changing patterns of family obligations, also play a part in influencing the wishes of individuals. In this complex and changing climate a number of important types of end of life decision have emerged in ethical debates that include:

1. The active termination of life by another person at the request of the individual who dies (made either contemporaneously, or at some point in the past by means of a 'living will'). This is often called 'active euthanasia'.
2. The active termination of life by another person without such an explicit request (although carers may judge this situation to be the course that the person who died might have chosen had they been able to do so).
3. Physician-assisted suicide, where a medical practitioner provides an individual with the means to end their own life.
4. The provision of treatment intended to relieve suffering in the knowledge that the treatment will also shorten life (an action involving 'double effect').
5. The withdrawal or withholding of life-sustaining treatment.

In this chapter ethical issues are explored by reference to research studies undertaken by myself and other colleagues over the past 15 years. These studies, firstly, have described the views of lay people reporting on the situations and preferences of their recently deceased relatives. Secondly, and more recently, my intention has been to discover the experiences of medical practitioners in this area of practice, as well as to compare UK doctors with those in other countries, some of which have more permissive legal systems, where comparable research has been done.

In choosing this focus, of course, a great deal about this subject is missed. Doctors are not the only ones involved in taking these actions; relatives, nurses and other carers are also sometimes involved. The views of relatives and their reports of deceased persons' wishes while alive may not be an adequate substitute for direct access to the views of people who approach the end of life, or indeed for the many opinion polls of general public views that have been done over the years. There is a vast literature that describes these other matters that would not be feasible to review here. It will become evident too that this is not, primarily, a discussion of the general ethical or philosophical principles that lie behind end of life decisions. I am not a philosopher or an ethicist, but a sociologist and therefore bring an empirical element to bear on this subject that is often not present in discussions that seek to elaborate underlying principles. At the same time I hope that it will be seen that these empirical investigations have numerous points of relevance for philosophical and ethical debates.

## Views of bereaved relatives and people approaching death

In collaboration with other researchers I was involved in organising and analysing a survey to investigate the views and experiences of relatives, friends and others who had known a sample of 3,696 people dying in 1990 in 20 areas of the UK. Our aim was to find out their views about the quality of care experienced by both the person who had died and by themselves, where relevant. The survey is, to date, the largest survey of this sort and provides the best evidence currently available for the preferences of a UK-based population of individuals facing death and caring for dying people concerning end of life decision making. The sampling covered all causes of death and enabled comparison between cancer and other illnesses that cause death, being to all intents and purposes a random and representative sample of deaths in the UK.

As well as a series of questions enquiring about the quality of care, the incidence of distressing symptoms and bodily restrictions and other matters, we took the opportunity of this survey to ask some questions about what we called 'euthanasia'. To be precise, these two questions were added to the survey:

- 'Looking back now, and taking (the deceased's) illness into account, do you think s/he died at the best time – or would it have been better if s/he had died earlier or later?'
- 'What about (the deceased)? Did s/he ever say that they wanted to die sooner?' and '(If yes) did s/he ever say that s/he wanted euthanasia?'

The study was published as four papers (Seale and Addington-Hall, 1994, 1995a, 1995b; Seale et al, 1997). What follows is based on a summary of these reports.

The study established for the first time the prevalence of requests for 'euthanasia' (based on what respondents understood by this term) and the relative role played in this context by pain as against dependency. The study also provided evidence that the 'slippery slope' argument against the legalisation of voluntary euthanasia may hold true for certain very elderly individuals vulnerable to subtle pressures to opt for death when they perceive themselves to be a burden on others. Evidence was also provided that contradicted the common argument that good quality health and social care, particularly that associated with hospice and palliative care, is associated with reductions in the incidence of euthanasia requests. Here are the details.

We showed that 28% of respondents and 24% of the deceased were said to have expressed the view that an earlier death would be, or would have been, preferable (Seale and Addington-Hall, 1994). In addition, 3.6% of the people who died were said to have asked for euthanasia at some point in the last year of life. We also examined factors that might have been causally related to the incidence of such requests and sentiments. We found that although much of the public debate about euthanasia concentrates on the role of pain, the experience of dependency was also a significant factor behind the request. We also found that this was a particularly important consideration for people dying with conditions that were not included under hospice and palliative care services, which largely provide for people with cancer. Additionally, although much of the public debate about the legalisation of euthanasia is influenced by religious considerations, religious faith was found to be largely insignificant in influencing the views of people actually facing their, or their relatives', deaths. This finding has important implications for the interpretation of opinion polls, since these are usually conducted on samples of healthy people who may be more willing to be influenced by ideology. By contrast we concluded:

When nearing one's own death … it appears that religious considerations and cultural influences fade into insignificance in the face of the overwhelming physical and emotional experience of suffering. (Seale and Addington-Hall, 1994, p 653)

## 'Slippery slope' argument

We then turned to an analysis that was to relate to the 'slippery slope' argument that is often used to oppose the legalisation of assisted dying. The argument is that such legislation would eventually fail to protect the interests of vulnerable elderly people who may experience subtle and not so subtle pressures to opt for euthanasia. In the light of demographic trends that leave more elderly people – particularly elderly women – living on their own or in institutional care towards the end of life than was once the case (see Seale, 2000), this issue is a serious consideration.

To address this argument, then, we examined some of the factors that influenced our respondents to say that an earlier death would have been desirable (Seale and Addington-Hall, 1995a). In particular, we were interested in comparing respondents who were spouses with other kinds of respondent, such as the (adult) children of the deceased. We found various indicators to suggest that spouses were more attached to the deceased person than any other group of respondents. Spouses were more likely than others, for example, to say they missed the deceased person, or that looking after the person had not been a burden even when spouses reported quite considerable labours of care. Spouses were less likely than others to feel that it would have been better if the person had died earlier and this held true even when we manipulated the statistics to control for differential levels of reported pain, distress, dependency and age in the deceased. Non-spouses (children and other relatives of the deceased, friends, neighbours and a few officials), on the other hand, were more likely than spouses to say an earlier death would have been better.

While this might be as one would expect (and of course it is equally possible that spouses' own judgements about the desirability of an earlier death were coloured by their own needs for companionship), this finding has some quite disturbing and systematic consequences for the very old. These people are more likely to be women because women live longer than men and tend to marry men somewhat older than themselves. Because of these underlying demographic trends older people were more likely to be cared for by people who, in retrospect, felt that it would have been better if the old person had died earlier. We found, too, that older people and women in particular, were more likely to be reported as having felt they themselves wanted to die earlier, even where they shared similar levels of symptom distress and dependency with others. This is consistent with the view that such people felt themselves to be a burden, or to have lives not worth living (although an alternative argument suggests that the sentiment is an expression of altruism towards those who feel obliged to care for them). It is not difficult to see the implications of this for the 'slippery slope' argument against the legalisation of voluntary euthanasia, which suggests a movement towards an involuntary state whereby a 'right' to die becomes a 'duty' to die.

## Role of hospice and palliative care

Finally, we turned (Seale and Addington-Hall, 1995b) to another argument commonly put forward by those who advocate the provision of hospice and palliative care services in place of the legalisation of euthanasia: that such good quality care can help people feel that their lives are worth living to their natural end, without recourse to euthanasia. Our findings suggest that the picture is in fact more complex. We found, even when we controlled for differences in reported levels of symptom distress and dependency levels, that people who received hospice care were, if anything, more likely to have respondents who felt that it would have been better if the people had died earlier. Investigation of the reported wishes of dying people suggested a similar picture, although here it was not possible to establish the time order of events, so it is possible that the reported wish had occurred before the episode of hospice care. In general, however, when we looked for associations between reports of good quality care (from whatever source) and the wish to die earlier, we found nothing to support the view that good care led to a reduced incidence.

## Planning for death

Finally, in the last paper in the series (Seale et al, 1997) we drew out the implications of a key difference on which people facing death differed: the degree to which they wished to plan for their deaths. People with cancer who wanted to plan in this way were more likely than others both to encounter hospice and palliative care services and be reported as having made requests for euthanasia. Hospice and palliative care appears to attract the kind of people who are also interested in considering euthanasia because such individuals are more able than others to accept and plan for their own deaths. It remains the case, of course, that such care may help people feel that euthanasia is not the best solution, but the argument for this view as yet remains unproven. We ended up questioning the contribution made by hospice and palliative care services to a reduction in the incidence of requests for assisted dying, even suggesting the opposite conclusion that such institutions foster a climate that actually encourages such a planned approach to death.

Subsequent research in Oregon, US, where physician-assisted suicide has been legal since 1998, has provided further evidence to support this view (Ganzini, 2004). Initially, there were concerns that physician-assisted suicide would be opted for disproportionately by poorer people in Oregon, by African Americans and by the uninsured without access to palliative care. In fact, the opposite is the case: in the first five years of legalisation no African Americans opted for physician-assisted suicide. It was largely chosen by people with higher levels of income and education, the vast majority of whom were enrolled on hospice and palliative care programmes.

Our findings then both established, for the first time, the incidence of requests of euthanasia in a random, representative sample of people at the end of life and demonstrated some of the factors that led to this request. On the way, we were able to shed light on some important ethical and policy debates that concern the legalisation of euthanasia. These debates included the claim that legalisation might lead to a slippery slope of obligation to die, as well as providing a deeper understanding of the relation between palliative care (largely restricted to cancer patients) and sentiments about the desirability of a hastened death.

## Medical practice

Although countries differ as to whether their legal systems allow for the practice of active euthanasia, or of physician-assisted suicide, these practices are known to occur in most countries. Either laws are not applied vigorously, or prosecutions fail to stick once public sympathy is recruited to support a doctor who has actively ended the life of his or her patient, or penalties for those convicted are mild, again reflecting a degree of sympathy for the professional dilemmas that can face doctors attending patients with terminal or otherwise debilitating illness. The discovery that some doctors are quite often willing to end patients' lives with active measures in spite of laws that prohibit this practice has, in Australia and Belgium, resulted in relaxations of the law in recent years (although in Australia this was confined to the Northern Territories only; and the law has since been nullified by actions taken by the national government). Here, the argument has been that if doctors are ending their patients' lives anyway, a wiser course would be to make the actions legal so that they can be exposed to a greater degree of public scrutiny. Thus surveys that seek to document medical actions in this area can have potentially important effects on arguments for legalisation. Although medical practices have been described in a number of countries, researchers have until recently been slow to investigate UK medical practice in this area. An exception is Ward and Tate (1994), who surveyed 273 general practitioners (GPs) and hospital consultants in one area of England, of whom 38 (14%) indicated that they had at one time or another 'taken active steps to bring about the death of a patient who asked them to do so'.

While this seems a high rate at which doctors appear to have been willing to contravene UK law, the figure is somewhat deceptive. It is well known that the wording of questions can influence the rates at which particular actions or opinions are expressed. In this case, all depends on what respondents thought the term 'active steps' actually meant. Clearly, the authors of the survey believed this to mean that the doctor had taken an action that was something like decisions 1 and 3 above ('active euthanasia' or 'physician-assisted suicide'). It is quite feasible, however, that decisions involving the withdrawal or withholding of life-sustaining treatment, or 'double effect' actions, were understood by respondents to be 'active steps'. Indeed, it is quite possible that no neutral question can be designed to elucidate the actual incidence of particular actions because of enduring problems with the variability of meaning in fixed choice questions, inherent in the process of questionnaire design. In these circumstances, it is much more illuminating to use such questionnaire devices to conduct *comparative* work, using the same questions across different groups of respondents – either people at different points in time, or practising in different parts of the world. Survey data of this sort then needs to be understood as providing estimates of *relative* rates at which decisions are taken, rather than absolute rates.

Additionally, surveys of doctors are an inadequate substitute for surveys of deaths. Different types of doctors deal with different types of patients. Ward and Tate (1994) found that GPs were more willing to contemplate active euthanasia, but such doctors see far fewer dying patients than do certain kinds of hospital consultant. A survey that adjusts for these differences between doctors is the most likely to give an adequate account of the proportion of deaths where various kinds of end of life decision are taken.

## International comparisons

In the Netherlands, where active euthanasia is legally permitted as long as certain safeguards are followed, surveys of this sort have been reported for a number of years, starting with a report by Maas et al (1991) published in *The Lancet*, which was based on interviews and mailed questionnaires to physicians who had attended people selected from a random sample of death certificates. This initial survey found that the most common forms of end of life decision to be carried out were those involving the withholding or withdrawal of life-sustaining treatment, or the provision of 'double effect' therapies, both of which accounted for 17.5% of Dutch deaths. A further 1.8% involved the administering of lethal drugs at the patients' request; 0.3% involved assisted suicide; and 0.8% involved 'life-terminating acts without explicit and persistent request', which, elsewhere in their report, the authors (unfortunately) translated as 'involuntary' euthanasia. The authors did not mean to imply by this term that these patients had been euthanised *against* their will, indeed the report states that "In more than half of these cases the decision had been discussed with the patient, or the patient had expressed in a previous phase of the disease a wish for euthanasia if his/her suffering became unbearable" (Maas et al, 1991, p 671). Nevertheless, critics have often pointed to these 'involuntary' cases in the Netherlands as evidence of a policy that contravenes the wishes of dying people.

It is instructive to examine the rates at which Dutch doctors reported 'ever' having practised euthanasia or assisted in a suicide: 54% reported having taken this action and GPs were particularly likely to say they had done (62%). This puts the finding of Ward and Tate (1994), reported above, into perspective since these authors found only 14% of UK doctors saying they had 'taken active steps' to end a patient's life. Although 14% may seem like a 'lot', the Dutch example shows that very large numbers of doctors (much more than in the UK) may report this, while the actual rate of euthanasia remains quite small when expressed as a proportion of deaths. If one were to use the Dutch proportions to extrapolate from Ward and Tate's (1994) figure to make an estimate of the proportion of UK deaths receiving such 'active steps', the estimate would be very small indeed.

The survey undertaken by the Dutch investigators involved a standardised questionnaire that has been translated into several languages, including English, and has been used by various teams of investigators to survey medical practice over time in the Netherlands (for example, Onwuteaka-Philipsen et al, 2003), in five other European countries (Deliens et al, 2000; van der Heide et al, 2003) as well as Australia (Kuhse et al, 1997) and New Zealand (Mitchell and Owens, 2003). The most recent of these surveys was done in the UK in late 2004 (Seale, 2006), providing for the first time an estimate of the extent of the main end of life decisions taken in UK medical practice that is comparable with a number of other European and other countries.

On the whole the survey (Seale, 2006) reveals that UK doctors report fewer decisions than doctors in other countries that involve the active termination of life (for example, active euthanasia at a patient's request where 0.16% of deaths were estimated to have involved such an action, or physician-assisted suicide where no cases were reported). Decisions to withhold or withdraw treatment, on the other hand, were more common than in a number of other European countries. Very few doctors (4.6% of 857 doctors) felt that UK law had inhibited or interfered with their preferred management of the patient on whom they reported. A culture of decision making informed by a palliative care philosophy (which prioritises comfort care and avoids taking active steps to end life) is therefore evident in UK medical practice. This emphasis is consistent with the UK having been centrally involved in the origination and development of palliative care as a medical and nursing specialty in the latter half of the 20th century.

## Conclusion and contemporary challenges

In many countries with advanced economies and highly developed systems of health care, there is periodic interest in the possibility of changes to laws that prohibit doctors from becoming involved in actively hastening patients' deaths. Such ethical and legal debates appear not to occur very much in poorer countries where, it may be guessed, medical care is less widely available and professional–client relations are less subject to public debate. In only a few countries though – and the Netherlands is the most well known example – is euthanasia more or less legal.

In the UK there has long been an active lobby to legalise euthanasia and there are periodic upsurges of public interest and parliamentary debate about this matter. At the time of writing, it appears that the issue is once again on the parliamentary agenda, this time because of a House of Lords proposed Bill to legalise physician-assisted suicide, which was accompanied by an inquiry report into the matter (House of Lords, 2005). Support for this kind of medical action is easier to gain than is support for active euthanasia (where a doctor, for example, administers a lethal injection). This is because the responsibility of the doctor is at one remove: the doctor's role is simply to provide the means for death without personally administering a lethal substance, a matter that is left to the patient themselves. Thus medical objections to involvement are somewhat reduced. Significantly, the British Medical Association dropped its long-standing objection to such a relaxation of the law in June 2005 (Sommerville, 2005). However, in adopting a neutral policy, rather than one that would involve campaigning for a relaxation of the law, the British Medical Association reflected some enduring concerns of its membership, all of which have been touched on in this chapter. These concerns are worth setting out below at the chapter's conclusion (adapted from Sommerville, 2005), as they provide a good indication of the key moral and practical issues involved:

• patients should be competent, informed and unpressured, able to change their mind at any stage;
• alternatives, such as good palliative care, ought to be available;
• doctors must have the right to object to involvement in such acts, without any prejudice to their careers;
• doctors who engage in such acts need special training that would focus, among other things, on dealing with the emotional consequences of such involvement.

These concerns draw attention to the continuing importance of avoidance of harms, while trying to ensure that a system is created that will not deny benefits to a small proportion of people who would otherwise endure intolerable levels of suffering. Given the range of ethical, moral and practical issues involved in any proposed legislation for physician–assisted suicide, both support and opposition are potential outcomes. Contemporary challenges are therefore likely to play a key part in any future developments.

## References

Deliens, L., Mortier, F., Bilsen, J., Cosyns, M., van der Stichele, R., Vanoverloop, J. and Ingels, K. (2000) 'End-of-life decisions in medical practice in Flanders, Belgium: a nationwide survey', *The Lancet*, vol 356, pp 1806-11.

Ganzini, L. (2004) 'The Oregon experience', in T. Quill and M. Battin (eds) *Physician-assisted dying: The case for palliative care and patient choice*, Baltimore, MD: Johns Hopkins University Press, pp 165-83.

Hausmann, E. (2004) 'How press discourse justifies euthanasia', *Mortality*, vol 9, no 3, pp 206-22.

House of Lords Select Committee on the Assisted Dying for the Terminally Ill Bill (2005), *Assisted Dying for the Terminally Ill Bill: First report*, London: The Stationery Office.

Kuhse, H., Singer, P., Baume, P., Clark, M. and Rickard, M. (1997) 'End-of-life decisions in Australian medical practice', *Medical Journal of Australia*, vol 166, pp 191-6.

Maas, P., Delden, J., Pijnenborg, L. and Looman, C. (1991) 'Euthanasia and other medical decisions concerning the end of life', *The Lancet*, vol 338, pp 669-74.

McInerney, F. (2000) '"Requested death": a new social movement', *Social Science and Medicine*, vol 50, pp 137-54.

Mitchell, K. and Owens, G. (2002) 'National survey of medical decisions at end of life made by New Zealand general practitioners', *British Medical Journal*, vol 327, pp 202-3.

Onwuteaka-Philipsen, B., van der Heide, A., Koper, D., Keij-Deerenberg, I., Rietjens, J., Rurup, M., Vrakking, A., Georges, J., Muller, M., van der Wal, G. and van der Maas, P. (2003) 'Euthanasia and other end-of-life decisions in the Netherlands in 1990, 1995, and 2001', *The Lancet*, vol 362, pp 395-9.

Seale, C. (1997) 'Social and ethical aspects of euthanasia: a review', *Progress in Palliative Care*, vol 5, no 4, pp 141-6.

Seale, C. (2000) 'Changing patterns of death and dying', *Social Science and Medicine*, vol 51, pp 917-30.

Seale, C. (2006) 'End of life decision making in UK medical practice', *Palliative Medicine*, vol 20, no 1, pp 1-8.

Seale, C. and Addington-Hall, J. (1994) 'Euthanasia: why people want to die earlier', *Social Science and Medicine*, vol 39, no 5, pp 647-54.

Seale, C. and Addington-Hall, J. (1995a) 'Dying at the best time', *Social Science and Medicine*, vol 40, no 5, pp 589-95.

Seale, C. and Addington-Hall, J. (1995b) 'Euthanasia: the role of good care', *Social Science and Medicine*, vol 40, no 5, pp 581-7.

Seale, C., Addington-Hall, J. and McCarthy, M. (1997) 'Awareness of dying: prevalence, causes and consequences', *Social Science and Medicine*, vol 45, no 3, pp 477-84.

Sommerville, A. (2005) 'Changes in the BMA policy on assisted dying', *British Medical Journal*, vol 331, pp 686-8.

van der Heide, A., Deliens, L., Faisst, K., Nilstun, T., Norup, M., Paci, E., van der Wal, G. and van der Maas, P. (2003) 'End-of-life decision-making in six European countries: descriptive study', *The Lancet*, vol 362, pp 345-50.

Ward, B. and Tate, P. (1994) 'Attitudes among NHS doctors to requests for euthanasia', *British Medical Journal*, vol 308, pp 1332-4.

# TWENTY

# Conclusion

*Susan McLaren and Audrey Leathard*

## Summary

This conclusion offers a summary of interrelated themes and ethical challenges that have emerged across chapters. Review of the content has identified five broad, emergent themes, the first of which explores ethical decision making utilising principles, models, professional codes and dialogue ethics in collaborative working across organisational boundaries and systems. A second theme, user–professional relationships and roles in the context of decision making, is focused on therapeutic relationships and virtuous practice, best interests, refusing treatment and end of life decisions, equity, resources and provider, professional and user relationships. A third theme, vulnerable people, summarises the challenges that can arise in charging vulnerable older adults for their care, vulnerability to loss of personhood, protecting the claims and entitlements of future people, child protection and protecting rights and welfare in research participation.

The theme of service users summarises the case for ethical involvement of users in health and social care and explores the benefits of services working together in relation to user involvement and outcomes. The exercise of choice, equity in access, balancing liberty and public safety and challenging ageism and discrimination are also explored from a user perspective. A final theme of governance and accountability links new forms of collaborative governance and their ethical justification, summarising current conflicts and challenges for governance frameworks in general and, more specifically, in relation to research. Our intention in writing this conclusion is to offer the reader both a summary and integrated synthesis of key themes and challenges; these themes are not intended to be comprehensive and there is much more in the chapter content that will repay exhaustive scrutiny by the reader.

## Ethical decision making

### Principles

Health and social care professionals can apply diverse theories (deontology, consequentialism, virtue ethics), rights, principles (autonomy, beneficence, non-maleficence, justice, fidelity, confidentiality), models and frameworks to inform decision making on ethical issues; legal precedents and professional codes of conduct are also relevant. All of the chapters in this text make reference to one or more of these approaches. In Chapter Two, Louise Terry reviews the application of ethical principles, for example autonomy, beneficence, non-maleficence and justice (Beauchamp and Childress, 2001), in a range of decision-making situations familiar to health professionals. However, in resolving ethical dilemmas, the point is made that sometimes principles can be in conflict and it is then necessary to determine which take priority. Limitations in the scope of the 'four principle view' have been discussed in the literature (Beauchamp and Childress, 1994; Seedhouse, 2002). In Chapter Five, Charles Campion-Smith also notes the conflicts between ethical principles that can arise in decision making and the role of virtuous professional practice in resolving these within the context of the therapeutic relationship between professional and service user (see page 286 below).

### Models

Does the use of models offer any advantages? The decision-making model of Jonsen et al (1998) outlined in Chapter Two is applicable to both health and social care, facilitating the collation of information that can impact on decision making, encompassing medical and social care indicators, personal preferences of the user, quality of life and contextual features. In contrast the framework suggested by Jeff Girling (Chapter Eleven) to provide a starting point for responding to ethical situations requires the professional to use intuition initially, moving on to apply values, rules and codes, principles/theories and finally to consider actions, analysing the likely impact of the decision (Newman and Brown, 1996). The use of models may help to clarify the process of ethical analysis, assist justification of decisions and procedural objectivity, but they seldom give a definitive answer to a dilemma (Chapter Two).

## *Collaborative working: professional codes, dialogue ethics, ethical discourse*

Codes of professional conduct can encompass ethical principles either explicitly or implicitly, but vary in the degree of guidance offered and can differ across professional groups, limitations acknowledged by Louise Terry (Chapter Two) and Jeff Girling (Chapter Eleven). Health and social care professionals and service users each see their rights and responsibilities through their own ethical codes, creating potential sources of tension. Current collaborative approaches to the delivery of care (interprofessional, interagency) emphasise that codes now have challenging organisational and political dimensions quite apart from the professional and this can impact on decision making. In the context of interprofessional working, Audrey Leathard (Chapter Seven) raises the issue of the extent to which information about service users can be shared across different administrative and professional boundaries without breaching confidentiality. A way forward could be to establish between groups, sectors and organisations working together an agreed code of interprofessional ethics reflecting the needs of all interested parties including users and professionals. 'Dialogue ethics', which offers a means of understanding and resolving moral disagreements that might arise within multidisciplinary teams, is advocated by Robert Irvine and John McPhee (Chapter Ten). The arguments in favour of this approach are that it emphasises mutuality, shared responsibility and accountability between professional disciplines and provides an alternative way of thinking about ethics (Bernstein, 1998).

Interagency working in a social care context can also raise challenges for confidentiality (sharing information), autonomy (risk and protection) and justice (unintentional discrimination), issues that are explored by Colin and Margaret Whittington (Chapter Six). Negotiation between professionals and users within a framework of interagency policies, obtaining a wider system view, joint planning that considers multiple perspectives in assessment and care planning, all offer a constructive way forward. With regard to working across organisational systems, Jeff Girling (Chapter Eleven) makes the point that a challenge facing ethics and management is to develop a form of ethical discourse grounded in management practices; again, a shared form of ethical discourse is seen as vital to achieve meaningful partnerships between systems of management and care delivery.

## Summary: contemporary challenges in ethical decision making

- Recognising barriers to effective interprofessional and interagency decision making on ethical issues.
- Critically appraising and utilising appropriate ethical principles, theories and models in conjunction with broader frameworks to assist decision making.
- Developing shared forms of ethical discourse and dialogue to achieve and enhance meaningful partnerships to the benefit of service users.

## Context of decision making: user–professional relationships and roles

### Therapeutic relationships, virtuous practice

The therapeutic relationship between professional and user, encompassing duty of care, based on ethical principles that embody trust, respect and reinforced by shared experience, lies at the heart of caring. An ethical practitioner will be aware of the therapeutic power the relationship has and will use this effectively. Charles Campion-Smith (Chapter Five) explores therapeutic relationships alongside the concepts of virtuous practice embodied in the virtuous practitioner as a moral agent. Virtuous practitioners can be characterised by the need to consider different viewpoints, recognise conflicts between ethical principles and weigh these in decisions, evaluate their own skills and knowledge in undertaking interventions, provide advocacy in access to treatments, and demonstrate probity in professional relationships with colleagues. Ensuring that in any discussions about treatment decisions information is presented free from personal bias is vital.

### Best interests, balancing conflicts

In Chapter Five, the conflicting responsibilities of professionals in terms of duty of care to the individual and need to balance this with obligations to the wider community are discussed. Considerations of beneficence need a clear view of what is in the users' best interests and the need to avoid unjustified paternalism. Jon Glasby, Helen Lester and Emily McKie (Chapter Seventeen) draw attention to the difficult situations that can arise in doctor–patient relationships in mental health care, regarding the implementation of community treatment orders (see page 247). These orders may result in certain circumstances in detention for enforced treatment, creating tensions for trust within therapeutic relationships and the risk that people may be driven away from services. The authors pose a challenging question regarding the stage at which the state has a right and duty to impose services on individuals for their own good and the safety of others (see also service users, page 248). In Chapter Sixteen, Keith Andrews explores best interests further in relation to users with complex disabilities, who lack the mental capacity to make decisions. Relevant to considerations of best interests are previously expressed views of the individual, advance directives, net benefit, futility and least restriction. Inherent in acting in best interests are the challenges and risks of imposing the values of the 'able-bodied'. In a broader context Louise Terry (Chapter Two) considers ethical dilemmas that can arise for users and relatives relating to justice and allocation of resources, where decisions may be made that are not in the best interests of all parties (see also governance and accountability, page 298).

## Refusing treatment and end of life decisions

Ethical issues relating to end of life decisions are explored by Keith Andrews (Chapter Sixteen) and in relation to euthanasia by Clive Seale (Chapter Nineteen). From 2007, advance directives "became rules with clear safeguards" (Chapter Sixteen, page 235), thus it will be possible for people to make advance decisions regarding treatment refusal, should the situation arise where they lack mental capacity. Inclusion of 'even if life is at risk' statements, duly signed and witnessed, will be needed to prevent life-sustaining interventions being initiated. With regard to end of life decisions concerning treatment refusal, the point is made that mentally competent individuals have the right to refuse treatment, illustrated by the case of a competent tetraplegic, whose request to have a ventilator switched off resulting in her death was supported in the courts. This contrasts with the situation in the well-publicised case of Dianne Pretty, who in the later stages of motor neurone disease sought protection for her husband to assist her suicide at a time of her choosing, and was not supported in the European Court of Human Rights, because assisted suicide is prohibited in current legislation. Louise Terry (Chapter Nine) makes the point here that the court were not persuaded that the right to life included a right to die, or that Article 3 of the 1998 Human Rights Act (the right not to be subjected to inhuman or degrading treatment) would be breached by the legislation on assisted suicide. However, in considering the arguments relating to the cases cited by Keith Andrews (Chapter Sixteen), the question is raised as to whether switching off the ventilator in the first case was assisted suicide?

Withholding versus withdrawing treatment at the end of life (most extremely in persistent vegetative states) also raises ethical dilemmas. In persistent vegetative states, a court directive is needed in England and Wales to withdraw but not withhold treatment. The point is made by the British Medical Association (BMA, 2001), that the decision-making process in both should be informed by the same criteria and that greater emphasis should be placed on the reasons for providing treatment, as opposed to its withdrawal. Requirements of 'best interests' apply to the decision making in cases where withdrawal of nutrition and hydration is considered in persistent vegetative states (see page 235). Louise Terry (Chapter Nine) draws attention to the decision by the courts in such cases, that Article 2 of the 1998 Human Rights Act (the right to life) "includes a positive obligation to give treatment if that is in the best interests of the patient, but not in situations where treatment would be futile" (see page 132).

In the context of euthanasia, Clive Seale (Chapter Nineteen) explores the dilemma of avoidance of harm, while trying to ensure no denial of benefits to people suffering intolerably. The benefits to the few need to be balanced against the interests of others through risks of creating a situation where older people might be pressurised into opting for euthanasia, 'the slippery slope' argument. Recent interest has focused, as part of the euthanasia debate, on 'physician-assisted suicide', where a doctor provides a person with the means to end their life. Clive Seale (Chapter Nineteen) points out that support for this is more easily gained than for active euthanasia, since the medical responsibility is at one remove. However, at their annual conference the British Medical Association (2006) voted to restore its long-standing policy of opposing euthanasia and physician-assisted suicide, overturning the previously held position of neutrality on assisted suicide.

## Equity, resources and provider, professional and user relationships

The finite nature of health and social care resources in relation to infinite demand are discussed in Chapter Two by Louise Terry. Public policies require priority setting, meeting targets and improving quality of care through evidence-based, cost-effective approaches, which, bearing in mind the nature of therapeutic relationships, can raise conflicts for health and social care professionals in relation to the utilitarian values of service delivery (Chapter Two). Mary Dombeck and Tobie Hittle Olsan (Chapter Twelve), in noting the inequities that can arise in access to health and social care through contexts defined by the person's ability to pay, comment that the evidence from behaviours of patients and consumers of health care is that relationships with providers are an important resource in a health care encounter, which has implications not only for organisational provider–user relationships, but also user–professional therapeutic relationships. Both patients and professionals can become depersonalised when patients are treated as goods and services, with negative consequences for therapeutic relationships (see also loss of personhood, page 180).

In relation to paying for services by older adults in residential and nursing care homes, Bridget Penhale (Chapter Thirteen) considers the role ambiguity and professional identity problems that can arise for managers and practitioners who acknowledge that the principle of equity is vital in paying for services. Perceived lack of clarity in aspects of managerial roles can create ethical dilemmas where personal and professional values can come into conflict, for example, in the completion of financial assessments and charging for long-term services. Development of transparent, consistent systems for financial assessment, aligned to the provision of training in ethics and financial aspects of managers' roles, offers a way forward (see vulnerable older people, page 290).

---

**Summary:** contemporary challenges in user–professional relationships and roles

- Balancing best interests of individual users with those of the wider community in health and social care decisions.
- Avoiding the imposition of values of the 'able-bodied' on individuals who lack mental capacity to make decisions.
- Removing inequities and injustice resulting from institutional structural arrangements that result in disparate care, services and depersonalisation of patients and professionals.
- Development of consistent transparent systems for financial assessment of users in residential and nursing home care.

---

## Vulnerable people

Brenda Almond (Chapter Fourteen) iterates a widely accepted moral and political principle, to protect the welfare and rights of those who are at a vulnerable stage of their existence and who are unable to protect themselves. The theme of vulnerability is examined below in relation to charging vulnerable adults for care; vulnerability to loss of personhood; protecting the claims and entitlements of future people; child protection; and protecting the rights and welfare of research participants.

## Charging for care: vulnerable older people

A key social policy issue relates to the extent to which people should pay for their own care needs in later life as opposed to care that is publicly funded (Chapter Thirteen). The implementation of the 1990 NHS and Community Care Act (DH, 1993) has resulted in financial assessment of an older person's ability to contribute to care costs and levying of charges for social care. Ethical dilemmas created by these events relate to conflicts between professional and personal values and role ambiguity for care home managers (page 191) and failure to treat all individuals equally, creating challenges for administrative justice. The latter result from the use of varying policies, procedures and practices between local authorities, and failure by some authorities to follow up charge avoidance and variations in the levels of charges for social care services. Bridget Penhale (Chapter Thirteen) suggests that the way forward lies in developing new systems for charging marked by transparency, openness and quality control. In order to ensure no disempowerment occurs in decision making, a need exists to acknowledge ethical principles and consider them within a human rights framework.

## Vulnerability to loss of personhood

Personhood as defined in terms of social and institutional relations is explored by Mary Dombeck and Tobie Hittle Olsan (Chapter Twelve); it is considered that a person is bound to social systems by rules that confer responsibilities and rights on them. Institutions then have obligations to these rights and responsibilities. Injustices can arise from inequities in resource allocation that result from structural arrangements in institutions in the US, increasing vulnerability to loss of personhood through depersonalising detachment from the system. For individuals with health care insurance, this can arise where their health care is governed by a corporate contract to which they were not a deciding party. Those receiving publicly funded care encounter bureaucracy and insecurity, while those reliant on charitable care are entirely detached from the system. Furthermore, conflicts can arise for health professionals when institutional policies clash with the interests of patients (page 179). The authors suggest that the way forward encompasses changes in health care policy and employing strategies to enhance the relationships between people and institutions, preventing loss of personhood through loss of voice (patients) and hearing (institutions).

## Protecting the claims and entitlements of future people

In the context of use of the new technologies of reproduction, vulnerability is explored in relation to the need to protect the claims and entitlements of future people conceived using these methods (Chapter Fourteen). Challenging questions are posed regarding the possession of rights by individuals to any available information about genetic identity or origins, and extension of the protections associated with adoption to assisted reproduction using gametes and whether or not valuable life experiences and/or a basic right is lost for children who, by virtue of their origins, are deprived of genetic links to carers, or to relationships with either or both of their parents. Further challenges are posed by the extent to which reproductive choice should be considered a private matter and a permissible exercise of autonomy, or be subject to legal regulation. Conclusions are that risks exist in guarding against the collapse of societies' moral responsibilities to vulnerable people and a failure to distribute the benefits of research equally.

## Child protection

David Hodgson (Chapter Fifteen) examines recent cases of abuse involving children that had different outcomes, reviews the issues that have arisen and their implications for reform, while the importance of not losing a broader perspective on ethical issues is emphasised. Insights from an analysis of childcare discourse are also used to explore selected aspects of the current UK reform agenda from a rights perspective. Conclusions are that ethical challenges exist in ensuring children's equal rights to privacy and physical and emotional integrity; maximising structures for their representation; challenging legal and policy contradictions that impact negatively on family support; and developing competence models in collaboration with children, families and professionals. In relation to legal contradictions and their negative impacts, in Chapter Nine, Louise Terry draws attention to the special protection that Article 19 of the United Nations Convention on the

Rights of the Child requires governments to take in protecting children from all forms of abuse. However, problems can arise from the interpretations of government Acts; for example, in the UK it has been recognised that the interpretation of 'significant harm' criteria in the Children Acts has resulted in over-representation of black children in care and failures emanating from "misunderstanding of different cultural mores" (page 129).

## Protecting rights and welfare in research participation

Research ethics committees implement additional policies and procedures to protect the rights and welfare of vulnerable groups, whose participation in research requires special consideration. Vulnerability can arise as a consequence of medical condition, social and economic disadvantage, dependent or unequal relationships, or other factors that impair decision-making capacity (Chapter Three). Particular concerns exist in relation to informed consent, notably to ensure that no undue pressures are placed on competent, vulnerable people to take part in research studies. It is also vital to ensure that vulnerable groups are not excluded from the potential benefits of research participation, since this raises the issue of discrimination. Anthea Tinker (Chapter Eighteen) explores these issues as they relate to vulnerable older adults, also noting the need to avoid covert pressures to take part in research and the potential barriers to research participation that can be created by protectionist gatekeepers. Furthermore, the exclusion of older people per se from clinical research trials raises particular concerns about them having the same rights and responsibilities as other age groups.

In a different research context, the participation in randomised controlled clinical trials by people in developing countries is raised by Susan McLaren and Robert Stanley (Chapter 3). Here, the dilemmas are that participants may not have at trial conclusion access to the most effective diagnostic and therapeutic methods, in accordance with World Medical Association (2002) principles, since standards of care do not approach those in more affluent countries and that a lack of international consensus exists on how to achieve justice in treating people equally in this respect. Finally, in relation to the participation of people with complex disabilities who lack mental capacity, in recordings made for a variety of purposes including research, teaching and audit, Keith Andrews (Chapter Sixteen) reviews the guiding principles that inform such decisions, including 'best interests' (page 230). Consideration of the alternatives that exist to showing the recording, direct benefits to the participant and benefits to other patients that accrue via the wider impact of the recording on clinicians, are all relevant in the case of audit and teaching.

---

**Summary:** contemporary challenges relating to vulnerable groups

- Risks in guarding against the collapse of societies' moral responsibilities to vulnerable people conceived using new reproductive technologies and a failure to distribute the benefits of research equally.
- Developing new systems for charging for long-term care that overcome administrative injustices and are marked by transparency, openness and quality control.
- Fostering and implementing strategies to enhance relationships between people, professionals and institutions that prevent loss of personhood.
- Responding to ethical challenges inherent in *Every child matters* reforms.
- Protecting the rights and welfare of vulnerable groups participating in research.
- Ensuring vulnerable groups and competent older people are not excluded from the potential benefits of research participation.
- Achieving international consensus on justice as fairness regarding the involvement of people in developing countries in controlled clinical trials.

---

## Service users

Developing and evaluating the quality of service delivery, facilitating service access and choice and at the other extreme imposing services, challenging ageism and discrimination all raise ethical issues that are selectively examined in the chapters by Jill Manthorpe and Martin Stevens (Chapter Eight), Audrey Leathard (Chapter Seven), Colin and Margaret Whittington (Chapter Six), Jon Glasby, Helen Lester and Emily McKie (Chapter Seventeen), Louise Terry (Chapter Nine) and Anthea Tinker (Chapter Eighteen).

### Case for ethical involvement

The ethical case for involving users in planning and delivery of current services, together with research evaluation to inform future developments, rests on considerations of respecting autonomy, maximising benefits (beneficence) and minimising harms (non-maleficence). The case for user involvement justified by Jill Manthorpe and Martin Stevens (Chapter Eight) identifies the need for services to be developed, delivered and evaluated in collaboration with the people whose lives are affected (respecting autonomy) and empowering users (beneficence, non-maleficence). Manthorpe and Stevens also review the frameworks and levels for user involvement in service planning, delivery and research. Ethical involvement requires transparency over current power imbalances and a move to sharing power and influence, which can require a reconstruction of professional roles and less emphasis on managerialism in public services. Challenges exist in funding service user involvement, avoiding consultation fatigue and achieving genuine equality in power sharing.

### Benefits of services working together: user involvement and outcomes

Currently, evidence that user involvement leads to improvements through enhanced service quality linked to measurable outcomes is limited. Such evidence would be powerful in justifying involvement from the perspectives of beneficence and non-maleficence. Audrey Leathard (Chapter Seven) explores the issue of who actually benefits from working together across health and social care services, noting the positive outcomes for users that have resulted from the implementation of support networks and the development of a membership organisation intended to enhance user involvement, aligned with other initiatives (Turner and Balloch, 2001). Further exemplars reviewed by Audrey Leathard (Chapter Seven) include collaboration between primary care trusts and social services, which have indicated changing attitudes of social services professionals in terms of listening to older people and enabling involvement in planning and reviewing service developments; early findings from the creation of care trusts also suggest that services can be improved for service users when local relationships are positive and a dynamic already exists to move forward. The need for continuing evaluations of partnerships between health and social care services to identify benefits to users is a challenge. Colin and Margaret Whittington (Chapter Six) also emphasise the challenges and ethical obligations inherent in measuring the impact of policies for user involvement within governance frameworks in terms of improvements in availability and quality of social care services.

## Exercising choice, equity in access, balancing liberty and safety

The exercise of choice by service users has been key to recent NHS reforms in the UK. Jon Glasby, Helen Lester and Emily McKie (Chapter Seventeen) identify risks that current proposals for reform contained within the Draft Mental Health Bill (DH, 2004) will deny users of mental health services access to the same principles and quality of care as other NHS patients. Although the Draft Mental Health Bill (DH, 2004) does address access to advocacy services and rights to refuse electroconvulsive therapy (ECT), specific concerns relate to the lack of opportunity for mental health service users to exercise choice through booking appointments and selecting certain treatment alternatives. Other issues raised by Glasby et al in Chapter Seventeen relate to the point that under the terms of the Bill, in severe mental health conditions, medical treatment can be provided to protect patients from suicide, serious self-harm, neglect of their health and safety and the safety of others. Specific concerns are that non–offending people with personality disorders could be detained indefinitely under certain circumstances. Furthermore, the impact of community treatment orders (CTOs) can mean that patients who fail to comply with attendance for medication under certain circumstances may be removed to a clinical setting to have medication administered.

In Chapter Nine Louise Terry reviews the legal challenges that can arise in relation to alleged breaches of Article 5 of the 1998 Human Rights Act (the right to liberty and security of person) regarding the detention of mentally disordered people. She makes the point that case law has established a precedent that the "burden of proving that the criteria for detention are no longer met should not rest on the patient seeking discharge" (page 134), and that the situation with overworked mental health review tribunals can lead to delays in discharge. Overall, these issues raise challenging questions for equity in user access to services, balancing individual liberty and autonomy with the safety of others and stages at which the state has the right and a duty to impose services.

## Challenging ageism and discrimination: older people

Anthea Tinker (Chapter Eighteen) reviews issues of fairness and justice in relation to service provision for older people, identifying issues of both positive and negative discrimination. Reasons for age discrimination are attributable to lack of resources, widespread ageism in society and the legacy of historical ageism in the welfare state

(Roberts et al, 2004). Evidence of discrimination relating to older people and the NHS has been disseminated (Gilchrist, 1999), yet recent publications by Help the Aged (2002) identify continuing problems in denying services to older adults, for example, breast screening and cardiac rehabilitation. The case is made by Tinker that ethically older people should be treated the same as any other group and have the same rights and responsibilities in society.

---

**Summary:** contemporary challenges relating to service users

- Achieving ethical involvement of users by provision of appropriate funding and training, creating opportunities for diversity in user representation and equality in power sharing.
- Evaluating user involvement in services linked to measurable outcomes.
- Achieving equity in user access to services.
- Balancing individual liberty and autonomy with public safety.

---

## Governance and accountability

### Collaborative governance

Governance is concerned with the implementation of policies through frameworks, which has ethical justifications and implications. It can be viewed as "a developing discourse of values and practices, ranging from the service level of clinical and social care governance to corporate and extra-corporate levels" (Chapter Six, page 89). New forms of collaborative governance have emerged through the implementation of interprofessional, interagency and partnership working involving users. Audrey Leathard (Chapter Seven) reviews the intentions encompassed in these new approaches that are to increase public participation and involvement in decision making, encourage active citizenship and overcome social exclusion, underpinned by considerations of justice, respect for autonomy and beneficence. Colin and Margaret Whittington (Chapter Six) also identify values of probity, efficiency, partnership, risk management, rights to high-quality services, honesty and transparency, justice and empowerment as intrinsic to governance.

## Challenges and conflict in new governance systems

Challenges exist where new forms of governance do not entirely replace the old and conflicts ensue, for example, in changing relationships between representative and participative democracy. New governance frameworks reinforce accountability across health and social care provision, requiring organisations and personnel to account financially and in other ways for services delivered to users. A strong driver for accountability lies in the demand for more efficient services that meet user needs and involvement in decision making (see pages 104-5). However, the emphasis placed on targets, procedures, outputs and demands generated by audit and regulatory processes can create an increased bureaucracy and a restrictive environment, for example in relation to the exercise of discretion and autonomy in professional decision making. Further challenges for accountability are created by the sheer complexity of interprofessional working, where different sectors work to different agendas and hierarchies of accountability also vary. Greater clarity is also needed in making new partnerships more accountable, for example between foundation trusts and primary care.

Colin and Margaret Whittington (Chapter Six) have reviewed the conflicts that can arise in interagency working, regarding sharing of information (confidentiality), risk and protection (autonomy) and anti-discrimination (justice). Other conflicts for governance can emerge where financial constraints hinder the provision of high-quality services and person-centred values conflict with organisational pursuit of, for example, standardised provision in social care. Jeff Girling (Chapter Eleven) also notes that the increased emphasis on regulation within governance has led to an increase in target-centred control, which is 'the polar opposite' of what works in achieving client-centred practice. He also suggests that managers, while accepting of the rights of government to implement policies, do have a degree of freedom in choosing how to act. It is suggested that this can be achieved by balancing the skills needed to implement roles with moral and social virtues that characterise healthy organisational cultures. The impact of such a culture at different organisational levels then not only benefits staff but also benefits patients, clients, partnerships and communities in a positive way.

## Research governance frameworks

In a different context, the intent in implementing the research governance framework (DH, 2005) across NHS-funded health and social care organisations has been to enhance the quality of research and development and to ensure a sustainable research culture (Chapter Four). Within a governance framework, the quality of research can be improved; rights, dignity and well-being of individuals protected and researchers are accountable for their actions. Furthermore, the move to involve users, carers and the groups representing them at all stages of the research process has been a step forward (see also user involvement, page 294). The ethical underpinning of the framework is founded on respect for dignity, rights, safety, well-being and valuing diversity. In addition, accountability, transparency and scientific integrity are also emphasised (Chapter Four).

Although much has been achieved by the introduction of governance frameworks, in practice, not everything has proceeded smoothly in the early stages. Concerns have been expressed relating to complexity of approvals processes, bureaucratic delays, increased research costs and a risk that researchers will engage in audit to avoid this. Susan McLaren and Robert Stanley (Chapter Three) suggest a need exists to reduce this complexity that has resulted in a constrained research environment. Inconsistent ethical standards, lack of transparency, together with coordination and efficiency of ethical review systems need to be reviewed.

**Summary:** contemporary challenges for governance and accountability

- Reviewing collaborative governance frameworks in health and social care to ensure accountabilities are clarified, and professional autonomy and discretion in decision making are not unduly restricted.
- Developing an ethical understanding of collaborative practice that addresses their complexities.
- Reviewing the application of risks and costs in governance that do not conflict with emancipatory values and codes.
- Evaluating the impact of governance frameworks on user involvement.
- Achieving more efficient coordination of ethical review, transparency and consistency of ethical standards within research governance frameworks.

## Envoi

This conclusion has identified many contemporary ethical and legal challenges, some emanating from new developments in health and social care; others are not new but continue to evolve. In diverse contexts, the exercise of autonomy, through its relationship to rights, is a common thread running through many chapters and poses powerful challenges. As Louise Terry concludes in Chapter Nine, despite many global declarations, the fact is that many have no access to health and social care or of obtaining their human rights. To paraphrase Thomas Paine (1737-1809)[1], "those who expect to reap the blessings of freedom must undergo the fatigue of supporting it". Can we meet these contemporary challenges in health and social care? Only time will tell.

## Note
[1] Taken from 'The American Crisis', n 4, 11 September 1777 (www.ushistory.org/Paine/crisis/singlehtml.htm).

## References

Beauchamp, T. and Childress, J. (1994) *Principles of biomedical ethics* (4th edn), Oxford: Oxford University Press.

Beauchamp, T. and Childress, J. (2001) *Principles of biomedical ethics* (5th edn), Oxford: Oxford University Press.

Bernstein, R. (1998) *The new constellation: The ethical–political horizons of modernity/post-modernity*, Cambridge, MA: The MIT Press.

BMA (British Medical Association) (2001) *Withholding and withdrawing life-prolonging medical treatment: Guidance for decision making* (2nd edn), London: BMJ Books.

BMA (2006) 'BMA votes to oppose assisted suicide', BMA Conference, Belfast (www.cbc.ca/cp/health/060629.html).

DH (Department of Health) (1993) *The NHS and Community Care Act*, London: HMSO.

DH (2004) *Draft Mental Health Bill*, Cm 6305-1, London: DH.

DH (2005) *Research governance framework for health and social care*, London: DH.

Gilchrist, C. (1999) *Turning your back on us: Older people and the NHS*, London: Age Concern.

Help the Aged (2002) *Age discrimination in public policy: A review of the evidence*, London: Help the Aged.

Jonsen, A., Siegler, M. and Winslade, W. (1998) *Clinical ethics* (4th edn), New York, NY: McGraw Hill.

Newman, D. and Brown, R. (1996) *Applied ethics for programme evaluation*, London: Sage Publications.

Roberts, E., Robinson, J. and Seymour, L. (2004) *Old habits die hard*, London: King's Fund.

Seedhouse, D. (2002) 'Commitment to health: a shared ethical bond between professions', *Journal of Interprofessional Care*, vol 16, no 3, pp 249-60.

Turner, M. and Balloch, S. (2001) 'Partnership between service users and statutory social services', in S. Balloch and M. Taylor (eds) *Partnership working: Policy and practice*, Bristol: The Policy Press, pp 165-79.

World Medical Association (2002) *Declaration of Helsinki, Ethical principles for medical research involving human subjects* (www.wma.net/e/policy/b3.htm).

# Index

# Also available from The Policy Press

## Negotiating death in contemporary health and social care

*Margaret Holloway*, *Professor of Social Work, University of Hull*

Once regarded as taboo, it is now claimed that we are a death-obsessed society. The face of death in the 21st century, brought about by cultural and demographic change and advances in medical technology, presents health and social care practitioners with new challenges and dilemmas.

By focusing on predominant patterns of dying; global images of death; shifting boundaries between the public and the private; and cultural pluralism, this book looks at the way death is handled in contemporary society and the sensitive ethical and practical dilemmas facing nurses, social workers, doctors and chaplains. The author brings together perspectives from social science, healthcare and pastoral theology to assist the reader in understanding and negotiating this 'new death'.

Paperback £18.99 US$29.95 ISBN 978 1 86134 722 0
234 x 156mm 224 tbc pages November 2007
BASW/Policy Press titles

## Understanding health and social care

*Jon Glasby*, *Health Services Management Centre, University of Birmingham*

This book provides a comprehensive and up-to-date analysis of both health and social care. It explores the origins of community health and social care and current services and looks specifically at partnership working; direct payments; independent living; anti-discriminatory practice; user involvement; and support for carers. Focusing on both health and social care in a time of increasing inter-agency working, the book includes a combined summary of current policy and practice dilemmas with useful theoretical frameworks.

With service user-focused case studies and reflective exercises to aid further study and analysis, this book is essential reading for anyone studying or working in health and social care.

Paperback £18.99 US$34.95 ISBN 978 1 86134 910 1
Hardback £60.00 US$80.00 ISBN 978 1 86134 911 8
240 x 172mm 224 tbc pages June 2007
Understanding Welfare: Social Issues, Policy and Practice series

# What is professional social work?
## Second Edition
**Malcolm Payne**, *Director of Psychosocial and Spiritual Care, St Christopher's Hospice*

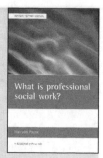

*What is Professional Social Work?* is a now classic analysis of social work as a discourse between three aspects of practice: social order, therapeutic and transformational perspectives. It enables social workers to analyse and value the role of social work in present-day multiprofessional social care.

This completely re-written second edition explores social work's struggle to meet its claim to achieve social progress through interpersonal practice. It includes practical ways of analysing personal professional identity and provides detailed analysis of current and historical documents defining social work and social care. The book also offers an understanding of how social workers embody their profession in their practice with other professionals.

Paperback £16.99 US$29.95 ISBN 978 1 86134 704 6
Hardback £55.00 US$75.00 ISBN 978 1 86134 705 3
234 x 156mm 232 pages July 2006
BASW/Policy Press titles

# Scandal, social policy and social welfare
## (Revised Second Edition)
**Ian Butler**, *School of Social Relations, Keele University* and **Mark Drakeford**, *School of Social Sciences, University of Wales, Cardiff*

*"This thought-provoking and enjoyable book offers a concise summary of historical trends and theoretical perspectives that helps the reader to see how the Climbie case, like other welfare scandals and inquiries, has both contributed to, and been shaped by, underlying seismic policy shifts."*
**Child and Family Social Work**

By examining the landmark scandals of the post-war period, including more recent ones, such as the Victoria Climbie Inquiry, this book reveals how scandals are generated, to what purposes they are used and whose interests they are made to serve.

Paperback £24.99 US$39.95 ISBN 978 1 86134 746 6
234 x 156mm 320 pages July 2005
BASW/Policy Press titles

## Social work and people with dementia
### Partnerships, practice and persistence
**Mary Marshall**, and **Margaret-Anne Tibbs**

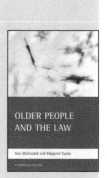

*"There has always been a shortage of material which gives enough attention to social work with people with dementia and this book fills an important gap. Mary Marshall and Margaret Anne Tibbs provide a comprehensive overview which will be invaluable for social workers practising in the changing world of health and social care provision."* **Jo Moriarty, King's College London, UK**

Paperback £17.99 US$29.95 ISBN 978 1 86134 702 2
Hardback £55.00 US$75.00 ISBN 978 1 86134 703 9
234 x 156mm 256 pages November 2006
BASW/Policy Press titles

## Older people and the law
**Ann McDonald** and **Margaret Taylor**

*"Older People and the Law is an important and timely reminder that changing demographics have considerable impact throughout every corner of society. The range of legal issues impacting on the lives of older people is wide. This book successfully draws together these diverse strands, and demonstrates both the limits of our current legal framework and the opportunities it presents for older people and their advocates."* **Michael Lake CBE, Director General, Help the Aged**.

Paperback £16.99 US$29.95 ISBN 978 1 86134 714 5
Hardback £55.00 US$75.00 ISBN 978 1 86134 715 2
234 x 156mm 184 pages November 2006
BASW/Policy Press titles

To order copies of this publication or any other Policy Press titles please visit **www.policypress.org.uk** or contact:

**In the UK and Europe:**
Marston Book Services, PO Box 269, Abingdon, Oxon, OX14 4YN, UK
Tel: +44 (0)1235 465500
Fax: +44 (0)1235 465556
Email:
direct.orders@marston.co.uk

**In Australia and New Zealand:**
DA Information Services, 648 Whitehorse Road Mitcham, Victoria 3132, Australia
Tel: +61 (3) 9210 7777
Fax: +61 (3) 9210 7788
E-mail:
service@dadirect.com.au

**In the USA and Canada:**
ISBS, 920 NE 58th Street, Suite 300, Portland, OR 97213-3786, USA
Tel: +1 800 944 6190 (toll free)
Fax: +1 503 280 8832
Email: info@isbs.com